Ferrozzi · Garlaschi · Bova
CT of Metastases

Ferrozzi · Garlaschi · Bova
CT of Metastases

Springer

Berlin
Heidelberg
New York
Barcelona
Hong Kong
London
Milan
Paris
Singapore
Tokyo

F. Ferrozzi · G. Garlaschi · D. Bova

CT of Metastases

With a Foreword
by P. Bassi

With 93 Illustrations in 140 Parts

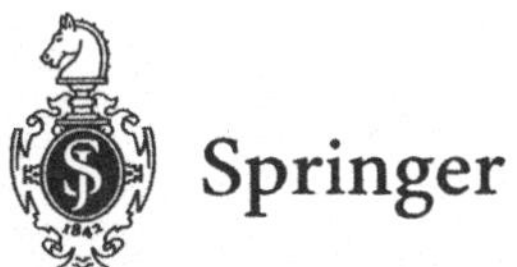

Springer

Dr. Francesco Ferrozzi
Istituto di Scienze Radiologiche
Universitá degli Studi di Parma
Via Gramsci 14
43100 Parma, Italy

Professor Giacomo Garlaschi
Istituto di Radiologia
Universitá degli Studi di Genova
Largo R. Benzi 10
16100 Genova, Italy

Dr. Davide Bova
Department of Radiology
Loyola University Medical Center
2160 South First Avenue
Maywood, IL 60153, USA

ISBN-13:978-3-540-65097-3   e-ISBN-13:978-3-642-59595-0
DOI:10.1007/978-3-642-59595-0

Translation from the Italian language edition: *La TC nello studio delle metastasi* by
Francesco Ferrozzi and Giacomo Garlaschi
© Springer-Verlag Italia Srl 1999
All Rights Reserved

Library of Congress Cataloging-in-Publication Data
Ferrozzi, F. (Francesco), 1957 – [TC nello studio delle metastasi. English] CT of
metastases / F. Ferrozzi, G. Garlaschi, D. Bova. p. cm. "Translation from the Italian
language edition: La TC nello studio delle metastasi by Francesco Ferrozzi and
Giacomo Garlaschi" – T.p. verso. Includes bibliographical references and index.
ISBN-13:978-3-540-65097-3 (softcover : alk. paper) 1. Metastasis – Tomography. I. Garlaschi,
G. (Giacomo), 1947 – II. Bova, D. (Davide), 1961 – III. Title RC269.5 .F4713 1999
616.99′40757 – dc21. 99-32320

Cover design: Erich Kirchner, Heidelberg
Typesetting: Fotosatz-Service Köhler GmbH, 97084 Würzburg

SPIN 10693782   21/3135-5 4 3 2 1 0

Foreword

It was with much pleasure that I agreed to present this monograph, authored by Francesco Ferrozzi, Giacomo Garlaschi and Davide Bova, on CT diagnosis of metastatic neoplasms.

The oncologic question, with its innumerable facets, is a daily reality for every radiologist, with a perpetual challenge of providing the clinician with ever more detailed information that is so essential in treatment planning. In particular, as stated by the authors, the changing philosophy in oncologic therapy – more aggressive and now routinely extended to metastatic tumors – has made it necessary for radiologist also to modify their perspectives and their practice.

The authors have approached the topic with an agile text, made particularly interesting by the additional documentation of variants and unusual aspects. The book combines a concise chapter on the biologic and pathogenetic aspects of metastatic diffusion with a discussion of the main modalities of metastasis (lymphatic, hematogenous, etc.), altogether providing extremely useful parameters to comprehend preferential sites of secondary spread in relation to the causative primaries.

The analysis of the structural aspects of metastases, where the morphology of lesions is accompanied by etiopathogenetic considerations, is of particular interest in relation to their differential diagnosis and to the possible identification of their origin.

The analytical discussion of each site of metastases, both rare and common, is organically and didactically organized and supported throughout by excellent images. More pragmatic aspects are addressed as well, as with the tables of differential diagnosis; the latter, by analyzing the crucial problem of the metastasis of unknown origin, suggest a simplistic but solid diagnostic path based upon analysis of anatomic, pathologic and etiologic criteria.

In conclusion, this is a lucid and accessible text, beautifully illustrated – the result of the authors' long experience in oncologic imaging – and of interest to anyone involved in the field.

Parma, May 1999 P. Bassi

Contents

Introduction 1

CHAPTER 1
Pathogenesis of the Metastatic Process 3

CHAPTER 2
Modalities of Metastatic Diffusion 5

Lymphatic Diffusion 5
Lymphangitic Infiltration 6
Hematogenous Diffusion 7
Neoplastic Seeding 8
Perineurial Diffusion 9
Neoplastic Thrombosis 10
Lepidic Diffusion 10

CHAPTER 3
Structural Features of Metastases 11

Calcified Metastases 14
Pseudocystic Metastases 20
Cavitation of Metastases 20
Cystic Metastases 22
Hemorrhagic Metastases 22
Lipoid Metastases 23
Infected Metastases 24

CHAPTER 4
Anatomical Sites of Metastatic Colonization 27

Classical Targets 27
Cerebrum 27
Lung 29
Pleura 37
Liver 39
Adrenal Glands 43
Peritoneum 45
Bone 48
Lymph Nodes 51

Rare Sites of Metastases   55
  Diencephalon   56
  Head and Neck   57
  Heart   60
  Breast   62
  Gallbladder   62
  Pancreas   63
  Spleen   65
  Gastrointestinal System   67
  Kidney   72
  Ureter and Bladder   74
  Female Genital System   74
  Male Reproductive Organs   76
  Soft Tissue   78

APPENDIX 1
Bizarre Metastases   81

APPENDIX 2
Differential Diagnosis Tables   83

References   91

Subject Index   97

Introduction

The therapeutic approach to neoplastic disease in metastatic phase has radically changed over the past decade. If in the past detection of secondary lesions almost invariably discouraged a potentially curative approach, presently metastatic disease, at least in selected cases, is managed more aggressively and addressed in a multidisciplinary fashion, with occasional excellent results in terms of both survival and disease control. This shift in therapeutic philosophy has determined an equal change in the diagnostic imaging field as well. Presently, in addition to the well-known concept of early diagnosis of cancer, there is renewed attention toward early diagnosis of both local and distant recurrence, in order to permit a timely and therefore potentially radical intervention. To this end, exact assessment of the anatomic extent of disease, in terms of number, sites, and morphostructural features, has become increasingly demanded by the referring oncologist.

In addition, the overall increase in survival rate of neoplastic patients and routine cross-sectional imaging follow-up have caused a parallel increase in detection of metastatic malignancies with less than typical aspects or in unusual locations. Also benign conditions, unrelated to the primary neoplastic disease, as well as new malignancies (relatively frequent in the clinical history of the oncologic patient) appear to be detected more and more often. In these problematic cases the differential diagnosis of metastatic lesions may be resolved only with the help of the pathologist.

Finally, thanks to improved technology and to more extensive clinical experience, a much wider morphologic and structural spectrum of pathologic and radiologic features of metastatic lesions has also been documented. These features depend primarily on the histology and biology of the primary tumor, which must in turn be the object of attention on the part of the radiologist. But these same features appear to be frequently the result of the therapy itself, therefore conveying prognostic information which may then be employed to modulate the pharmacologic and radiotherapeutic attack along the course of the primary disease.

In this scenario we have described, and, when possible, analyzed the polymorphous aspects of metastases on CT, their modalities of diffusion, structural features, and their sites of elective colonizations, placing particular attention on less than usual behaviors or localizations.

CHAPTER 1

Pathogenesis of the Metastatic Process

Metastatic diffusion represents the final result of a complex series of events related both to the host and to the tumor, strictly interrelated and all equally essential. The incomplete realization of one or more of these phases or events may indeed prevent the formation of a metastasis altogether [1].

Local invasion and angioneogenesis represent the beginning hallmark of the process. Proliferating neoplastic cells infiltrate along and through various extracellular matrices (basal membrane, interstitial stroma) systematically following three biochemical and biologic steps. These steps are cellular *adhesion, proteolytic degradation* of the substrate, and *passage* of the tumoral cell through the degraded substrate [2]. Paracrine chemotactic factors, autocrine motility, several growth factors and catabolites of the enzymatic proteolysis are all involved in the genesis of the phenomenon [3]. Only when the tumoral population reaches a critical volume (generally 1 – 2 mm in diameter), are angioneogenetic events also observed. The secretion of molecules suppressing homeostatic inhibitory factors, together with the *production* of stromal and tumoral angiogenic factors, causes proliferation of endothelial cells, especially in the post-capillary venules. This proliferation may occur at rates between 20 and 2000 times higher than the normal reproductive speed [4].

The subsequent *intravascular colonization* is facilitated by the typical histologic structure of the angioneogenesis, characterized by discontinuity and fenestration of the endothelium, which therefore allows tumoral migration into the systemic circulation [5]. The cells that penetrate the bloodstream, whether alone or in aggregates, are predominantly destroyed by circulating macrophages and by reticulo-endothelial cells in general. Only a minimal proportion (less than 0.01%) successfully initiate a proliferative cycle and create a new tumoral colony [1].

In turn, the arrest in distant organs of cellular aggregates occurs by cohesion to fibrin and platelets or, alternatively, to specific receptor sites. Different neoplastic types display different factors and modalities of adhesion, with different preferential metastatic organs [6]. This probably represents a fundamental mechanism in the determination of selective tropism of metastatic localizations [5].

The subsequent *extravascular diffusion* of the tumoral cells is obtained by means of exposure and proteolysis of the basal membrane, after cellular adhesion to the endothelium. Adhesion may further be favored by conditions that alter the structural integrity of the endothelium, such as trauma, inflammation, and fibrosis [1].

Growth of the cellular colony and implantation of the tumoral metastasis are permitted by secondary angioneogenesis, the final link in a chain of events [4]. Again, the previously evoked autologous tumoral factors and elements derived from the local microenvironment concur to create favorable conditions to colony development. Local factors in particular may represent ulterior elements in characterizing selective organ tropism of metastases [3, 6].

CHAPTER 2

Modalities of Metastatic Diffusion

In addition to the specific immunologic and biochemical tropism of a given neoplasm, its usual routes of diffusion are the single most important predictor of metastatic sites. These routes are often directly related to the histology and site of origin of the malignancy itself; hence, the need to acknowledge, in addition to the main metastatic routes and the typical primary and secondary "filter" organs, also those factors specific to each neoplasm which may justify metastatic disease in organs which are only apparently atypical [7]. For example, the existence of an accessory venous system, such as the venous plexus of Batson, deprived of valves and freely communicating with the main venous circulation, accounts for vertebral, pelvic, and upper femoral metastases from prostatic cancer, despite the absence of visceral involvement [1]. An analogous mechanism has been invoked to justify dorsal and cervical vertebral metastases without pulmonary involvement from breast cancer, or cerebral metastases from bronchogenic carcinoma, in which case direct colonization of vertebral veins takes place through the posterior bronchial vein [7].

Although metastatic diffusion is a complex and variable process, most tumors display typical patterns of spread according to the originating histotype.

■ Lymphatic Diffusion

Rigid differentiation among the different routes of metastatic diffusion is not possible, due to the interdependency of the various mechanisms involved. Epithelial malignancies, however, preferentially disseminate through the lymphatic system [7]. The neoplastic cells, once their intercellular adhesion is lost, penetrate the lumen of local lymphatic vessels and migrate, through afferent lymphatics, toward the marginal sinus of a lymph node. Although these same tumoral cells may be eliminated by the immunologic system, more often they undergo local proliferation, initially within the lymph node and subsequently breaching the capsule, the latter taking place earlier in biologically more aggressive tumors [1]. Violation of the capsule leads to invasion of the surrounding tissues and organs, with reproduction of the growth modalities already employed at the primary sites. Although tumoral diffusion tends to involve contiguous nodal stations and chains in an ordinate fashion, the presence of anastomoses between lymphatics and veins, along with direct invasion of capillaries, maylead to colonization of distant lymphatic chains [7].

As a rule neoplastic invasion of the lymphatic vessels leads to obstruction of the lymph circulation and, at least in early phases, to collateral circulation. When the latter vicarious mechanism ultimately fails, the lymph flow may invert its direction, producing distal satellite metastases in anomalous locations. This chain of events often lies behind the production of dermal localizations from melanomas or breast carcinomas [1, 8]. Obstruction of the internal thoracic lymphatic pathway may cause retrograde metastatization to the liver through the lymphatics of the recti abdomini and the falciform ligament [7]. In an analogous fashion gastric and pancreatic carcinomas metastasizing to the celiac and para-aortic lymph nodes may cause retrograde involvement of the iliac and inguinal chains, with a progressive centrifugal reduction in size of the diameter of metastatic nodes [7, 9, 10]. This same mechanism has also been advocated to explain contralateral localizations, such as the axillary one in breast carcinomas or the latero-cervical localization in head and neck tumors.

The most advanced picture of lymphatic metastatization is produced when the cisterna chyli and the thoracic duct are occluded by tumor, an event that can be encountered in up to 37% of cases of systemic disease. These are the patients who present with extensive neoplastic diffusion with involvement of the retroperitoneal space, the thoracic wall and the major central nodal stations of the groin, pelvis, abdomen, axilla, and neck [7].

■ Lymphangitic Infiltration

Lymphangitic infiltration is a massive metastatization of the lymphatic bed of a single organ, often associated with marked desmoplastic reaction [5]. According to recent studies, the initial pathologic event appears to be a synchronous involvement of the capillary bed, occasionally even preceding the lymphatic invasion itself [11]. Epithelial tumors, and in particular breast, gastric, pancreatic, and lung cancers (Fig. 1), are the most frequently responsible neoplasms.

The classic anatomical site of this modality of spread is the *lung*, where lymphangitic infiltration accounts for approximately 8% of all secondary neoplasms [12]. It typically presents with bilateral lesions (especially when not originating from the lung or breast), marked by irregular thickening of the interlobular septa, and of

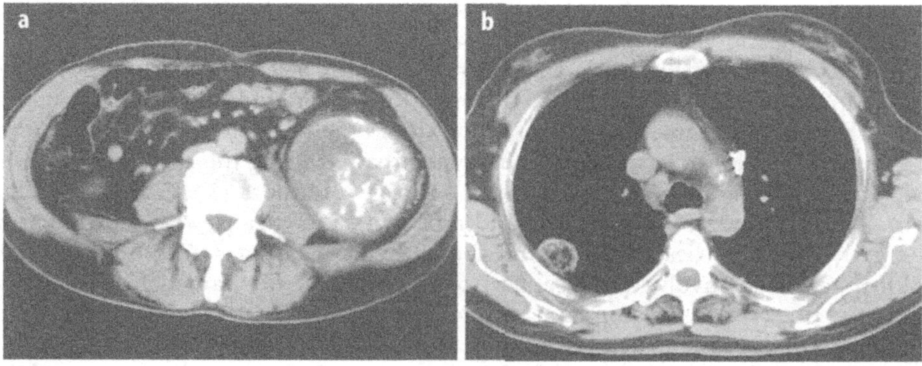

Fig. 1. a Diffuse metastatic involvement of the lower pole of the left kidney secondary to mucoid *adenocarcinoma of the sigmoid colon*, with evidence of multiple coarse foci of calcification. **b** Subpleural metastasis, from a *retroperitoneal mixoid liposarcoma*, demonstrating several areas of negative HU values, as expression of the lipoid nature of the neoplasm

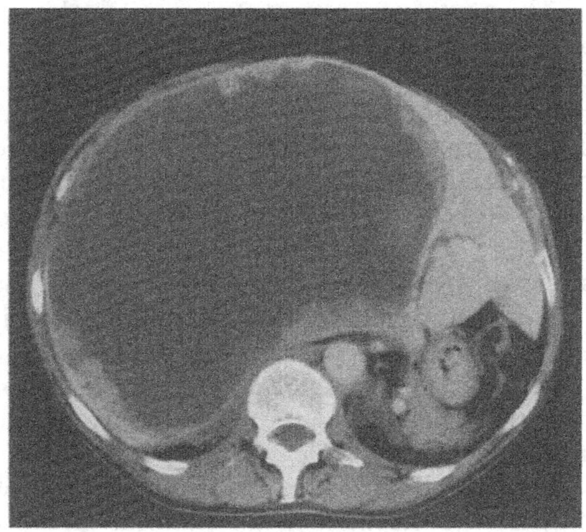

Fig. 2. Voluminous hepatic metastasis from a *bilateral serous cystadenocarcinoma of the ovary*. The lesion appears frankly cystic with evidence of several nodular and papillary solid formations

the peribronchial and perivascular as well as the subpleural septa. The septal thickening may occasionally have a micronodular appearance [13].

Lymphangitic diffusion to a *hollow organis* is, on the other hand, generally secondary to highly aggressive and anaplastic carcinomas. In these cases the massive invasion of the lymphatic vessels elicits an aggressive desmoplastic response, with marked parietal thickening and stiffening, flattening of the mucosal plicae and minimal, if any, ulcerative changes [7]. Occasionally, the infiltrates may appear at CT as hypodense sub- or intramural bands, with only mild contrast enhancement. Such an aspect, occasionally termed as "metastatic linitis plastica" (Fig. 2), is most often seen with primaries originating from the breast, pancreas, or bladder [14, 15].

With the exception of lymphomas, lymphangitic involvement has also been rarely reported in *solid organs* such as the liver. Here the tumoral growth occurs mostly along the perivascular spaces, with dilatation of the lymphatic ducts, infiltration of the periportal spaces and secondary fibrosis [16].

■ Hematogenous Diffusion

Hematogenous diffusion is facilitated by the deficient development of the vascular endothelium within the tumor and generally takes place through venous invasion at the level of the capsule or in the peripheral portion of the neoplasm. The distribution of the tumoral emboli appears somewhat casual, but each histologic type demonstrates one or more preferential targets of metastatic diffusion [2, 6].

The main hematologic route of diffusion is through the *systemic circulation*. Beyond the step of venous penetration, the first filter is represented by the pulmonary capillary bed [5]. Melanomas and renal, thyroid, adrenal,testicular, head and neck, and bony neoplasms all encounter the lung as their first systemic filter [7]. The occurrence of distant metastases in the absence of synchronous pulmonary involvement may be explained by the presence of arterio-venous shunts that allow bypassing of the pulmonary capillary network [7].

The *portal venous system* essentially drains the gastro-enteric tract with the liver as the primary filter. Systemic metastases to other organs generally necessitate prior diffusion to and through the lung [6]. Detailed knowledge of the specific vascular territories and their pathways is therefore extremely helpful in the research of early signs of metastatic diffusion. For example, the venous drainage of the inferior third of the rectum is a tributary of the inferior vena cava, via the inferior hemorrhoidal veins, and can therefore be the origin of metastases to the lung. Tumors of the upper two thirds of the rectum alternatively metastatize electively to the liver, through the superior mesenteric vein and the portal venous system [7].

Neoplastic emboli released from the lung into the *pulmonary veins* can be filtered by any vascularized parenchyma. Organs and tissues with dual vascular supply (liver, lung) or with arterio-venous shunts (bone, adrenal glands) demonstrate areas in which blood circulation slows down and the endothelial area increases remarkably, offering favorable conditions for the neoplastic implantation [1, 6].

Retrograde diffusion, in the presence of obstruction of main venous pathways, may be the mechanism for tumoral spread to atypical sites. This is the case, for example, for isolated vulvar or vaginal metastases in patients with obstruction of the left renal vein, subsequent retrograde neoplastic embolization of the left gonadal vein, and diffusion to the utero-vaginal venous plexus. In male patients the same process takes place through the pampiniform plexus, ultimately leading to epididymal and spermatic cord metastases [1, 7].

Other well-described mechanisms of hematogenous diffusion are related to variations in intrathoracic or intra-abdominal pressure which may temporarily invert the direction of flow in the paravertebral plexus of Batson. Batson's plexus is a complex venous system, devoid of valves, which is anastomosed with the inferior and superior caval system, as well as with the azygos–hemiazygos system. The renal veins may occasionally present communication in the retroperitoneum with the azygos system, thus accounting for the peculiar ability of some left renal and adrenal tumors, as well as prostatic or other pelvic neoplasms, to skip altogether the classic caval, portal, or pulmonary diffusions and metastatize to other districts [7].

■ Neoplastic Seeding

Neoplastic seeding is the classical modality of diffusion to and through mesothelium lined cavities (pleura, pericardium, and peritoneum) and is exemplified by the peritoneal extension of ovarian carcinomas [7]. Other mucin-producing malignancies, most often from the stomach, colon, pancreas, and gallbladder, may employ this route of metastatization as well, therefore gaining early access to the abdominal and thoracic serosal spaces [1]. The mesothelial lining of these cavities appears particularly vulnerable to violation by tumoral cells, which proliferate producing flat or nodular lesions, which in turn shed large numbers of cells within the serosal cavity. Both tumoral implants and cellular shedding elicit an exudative response and the effusion in turn favors further diffusion of neoplastic cells within the cavity. This, with the occasional permeation and obstruction of the lymphatic vessels, overall augments the malignant process. In the peritoneum this becomes particularly apparent, thanks to the preferential direction of flow of the ascitic fluid, determined by gravity, cyclical pressure variations, intestinal peristalsis, and mesenteric anatomy. Preferential sites of tumoral seedings are regions of decreased or arrested flow such as the right subphrenic space or the pouch of Douglas [7].

Within the peritoneum, a particular event is the so-called *pseudomyxoma peritonei*, a term considered obsolete by some authors. This is the result of diffuse peritoneal and omental colonization (through rupture or direct metastatic implants) by a low-grade mucinous epithelial neoplasm, originating from the ovary, appendix, pancreas, and gallbladder [7]. Cases secondary to tumors of the uterus, urachus, or omphalo-mesenteric duct have also been reported in the literature [17]. The macroscopic appearance is one of massive peritoneal infiltration by a gelatinous, occasionally loculated, mass which may solidify the entire abdomino-pelvic cavity [18].

Somewhat less frequently, neoplastic seeding takes place in the pleura or the pericardium. Lymphatic permeation is considered a fundamental part of the process in these districts [7]. With the exception of the most dependent regions, there are no preferential sites of localization.

An analogous process may also take in the central nervous system where tumoral diffusion may invade the cerebral and spinal leptomeninges or the ependyma that lines the ventricles [1]. For example, the medulloblastoma, from its primary cerebellar location, may colonize the epidural spaces, giving rise to the well-known "drop metastases." Secondary tumors of the central nervous system may similarly display leptomeningeal diffusion through invasion of the dural venous sinuses or, after gaining access through the intervertebral foramina, through perineural or perilymphatic extension [7].

Neoplasms of the female genital tract may gain access to the salpinges, through the endometrial cavity. This process is probably favored by the scant production of mucus and the absence of saprophytic bacteria, known to exert a protective action, in post-menopausal women [1].

Drop colonization has also been described in the urinary system, again probably favored by the sterility of urine and the relative paucity of mucus. Papillary tumors in the distal ureter and in the bladder, secondary to primaries of the renal pelves, are a not uncommon occurrence, even accounting for the frequent multifocality of urothelial malignancies [1, 7].

Metastases to joint spaces are, on the other hand, extremely rare, probably because cartilage possesses a protective low-weight protein molecule which inhibits proteases and neoplastic angioneogenesis [1].

■ Perineurial Diffusion

The term perineurial diffusion refers to the ability of selected neoplasms to propagate toward distant sites along preformed routes constituted by neural bundles, without involvement of the intermediate nodal stations or other organs [1]. It is a phenomenon of great clinical importance since it affects both prognosis and therapeutic choices by excluding radically curative surgery [19].

From the pathologic point of view, this process consists of direct tumoral invasion, with centripetal growth along the endo- and perineurial spaces. This process causes a concentric increase in diameter of the nervous trunk, with secondary erosion and enlargement of pertinent neural canals and foramina [7].

The relatively high resistance to neoplastic invasion of the axonal fibers is responsible for subtle, late, and often aspecific or atypical symptoms; therefore, the clinical findings may be entirely negative well ahead into the biologic history of the neoplastic process.

Otolaryngologic neoplasms, particular salivary adenoid-cystic carcinoma, cylindromas, squamous cell carcinoma of the oral, nasal, and paranasal cavities, lymphomas, recurrent cutaneous epitheliomas, and the neurotropic variant of melanoma, are the histologic types most often exhibiting this pattern of metastatic spread [7, 20].

Cranial nerves, V and VII in particular, are among the most frequently involved structures. The numerous anastomoses between the fibers of these two nerves explain the frequent cross-metastatization [21].

■ Neoplastic Thrombosis

Massive endovascular diffusion is typical of some tumors (renal cell and hepatic cell carcinomas, adrenal carcinoma, uterine leiomyosarcoma) which display the tendency to shed multiple neoplastic emboli. These emboli in turn proceed along the venous system, causing vascular occlusion and ultimately venous thrombosis [7]. The pathogenesis is probably related to aggregating factors secreted by tumoral cells [5].

From the kidney, the process can easily extend through the ipsilateral renal vein into the inferior vena cava and up to the right atrium. The liver, the portal system, the hepatic veins, and again the inferior vena cava are the targets of tumoral progression [7]. Detection of neoplastic thrombosis, typical of these neoplasms, is an extremely helpful clue in differentiating between primary and secondary lesions.

■ Lepidic Diffusion

Lepidic diffusion is an uncommon modality of pulmonary metastatization, similar from the pathogenetic standpoint to the pattern of growth of bronchiolo-alveolar carcinoma. It is a permeative tumoral proliferation through intact alveolar walls, probably through cellular diapedesis, analogous to what is seen in inflammatory exudative processes [7]. The diffusion takes place along the thin spaces of the alveolar stroma which, at least in the initial phase, remain intact. The result is represented by massive infiltration of the alveolar walls, with appearance of air-bronchograms and parenchymal consolidation, non-segmental in distribution [13]. However, the picture is rarely so extensive as to be macroscopically apparent, with a frequent discrepancy between the radiologic and pathologic findings. Adenocarcinomas, especially arising from the pancreas and bowel, are more frequently responsible for this pattern of metastatization [2, 20].

CHAPTER 3

Structural Features of Metastases

The structure of metastases exhibits a high degree of variability in relation to the histologic and biologic characteristics of the primary tumor, to the cytologic architecture of the single focus and of the surrounding tissue host, as well as to the degree of vascularization and to the dimensions of the metastasis itself.

Histology is one of the fundamental parameters determining the appearance of metastatic lesions. For example, differentiation toward secretion with a significant extracellular component or the presence of specific cells, such as adipocytes or osteoblasts, has an obvious effect on the attenuation values of the lesion (Fig. 1) [23]. Especially in the mixed or complex histologic types, awareness of the close relationship between the histopathologic appearance and the CT findings is very important (Fig. 2).

The grade of cellular anaplasia is directly related to the rate of cellular growth and often to the degree and character of therapeutic response. Similarly, regressive phenomena, such as cystic or mucoid degeneration, dystrophic calcification, and hemorrhage, are all primarily related to the histology of the primary tumor (Fig. 3) [23].

Tumoral *cytologic architecture* also plays an important role. It may indeed affect not only the structural appearance (highly cellular tumors appear hyperdense at CT, Fig. 4), but it may also influence the pattern of growth (expansile or infiltrating) upon the anatomic substrate (Fig. 5) [24]. Additionally, the host tissue may itself react to the tumor with edema or a desmoplastic response, therefore changing its intrinsic densitometric characteristics at CT (Fig. 6) [23, 25].

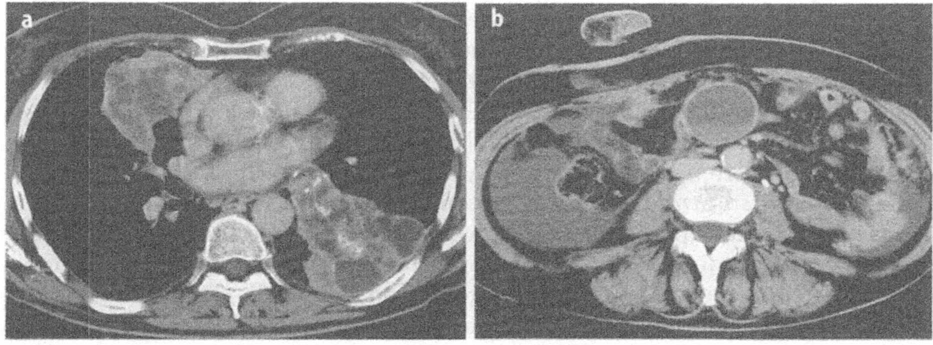

Fig. 3. a Large bilateral pulmonary lesions, secondary to a mucoid adenocarcinoma of the stomach currently under chemotherapy. The structure of these masses is characterized by involution with mucoid, necrotic, and calcific components. **b** Hemorrhagic metastasis to the mesentery, from a *gastric leiomyosarcoma*, with uniformly thickened walls and hematocrit level

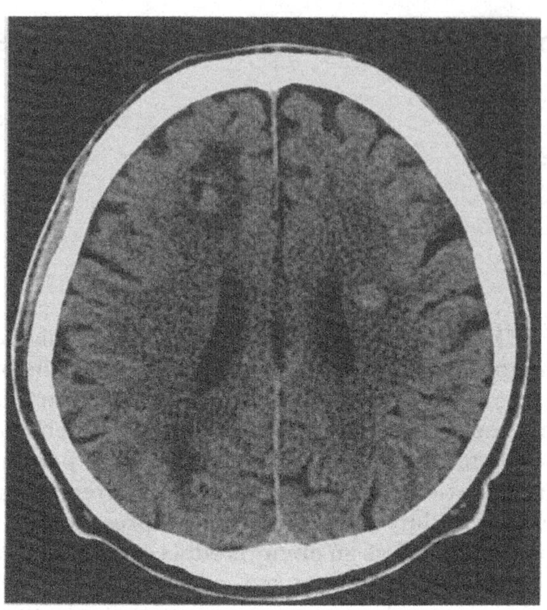

Fig. 4. Cerebral metastasis, midly hyperdense at non-enhanced CT examination, secondary to *small cell lung cancer*

The degree and type of *vascularization* of both the tumor and the surrounding organ are probably the most important factors affecting the CT appearance of metastases, thanks also to the central role that iodinated contrast material has achieved in generating contrast gradients between normal and pathologic tissues. Particularly in those districts with a dual vascular supply, such as the liver, administration of intravenous contrast results in different sensitivity in detecting lesions. Additionally, the lesions themselves may demonstrate different structural features in the sequential arterial and portal venous phases (Fig. 7). The enhancement patterns of neoplastic lesions may exhibit the same degree of variability in relation to the peculiarity of the tumoral vascularization. Enhancement may be characterized as global or segmental, centripetal or peripheral, homo or heterogeneous (Fig. 8). The majority of hepatic metastases are however hypodense due to their relative hypovascularity in comparison to the surrounding hepatic parenchyma [23].

As already stated, the *dimension* of the neoplastic focus represents a critical factor in relation to the tumoral metabolic necessities. Above a critical volume, particularly in those tumors exhibiting a high mitotic index, evolution toward necrosis is frequent, most often centrally, where hypoxia is more likely (Fig. 9) [23, 24].

The *anatomic substrate* of the host organ also deeply affects the appearance and the possibility of detection of metastatic lesions. For example, the pulmonary parenchyma, with its predominantly gaseous structure, represents an optimal anatomic background upon which even millimetric lesions are easily discernible (Fig. 10). Analogously, the alteration or destruction of the blood-brain barrier is responsible for the extravascular pooling of contrast medium, resulting in the marked enhancement typically seen in cerebral metastases (Fig. 11) [25]. On the other hand, the inherent hypervascularity of the spleen and kidney, despite offering important information in the absence of the expected parenchymal enhancement, obviously

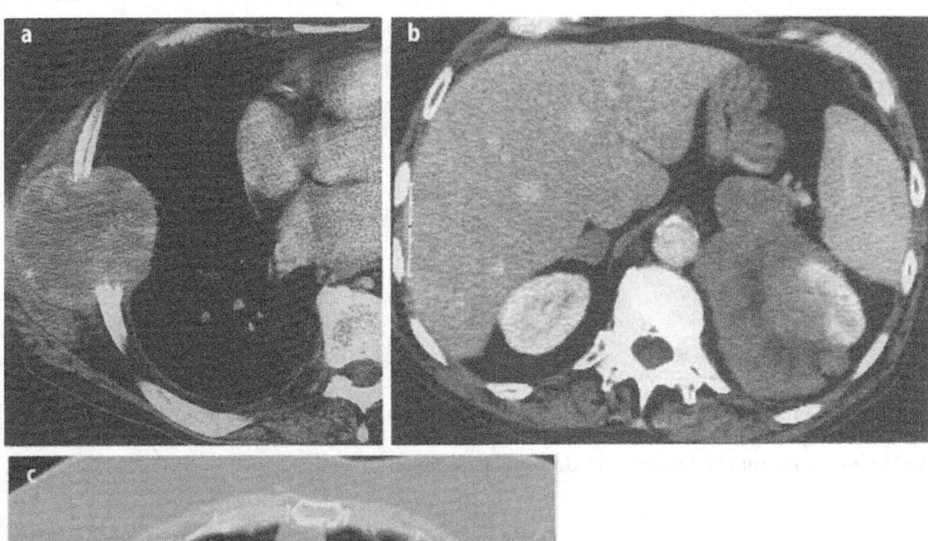

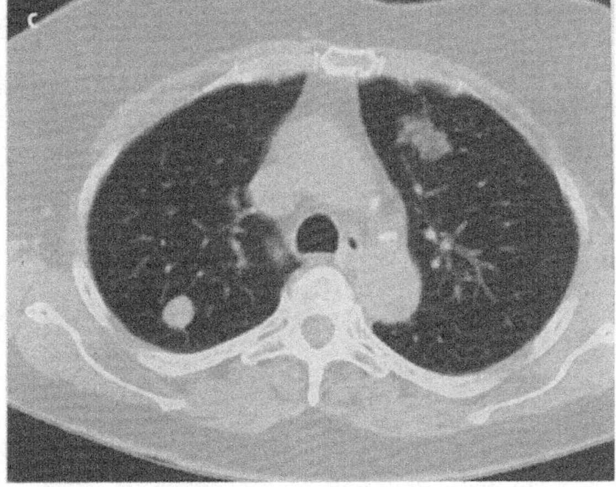

Fig. 5a–c. Patterns of metastatic growth in different anatomic substrates. **a** Espansile growth of a metastasis from *clear cell renal carcinoma,* causing erosion of the bony structure of the rib and subsequent substitution by soft tissue with a necrotic component. **b** Infiltrating lesion, from an *epidermoid carcinoma of the lung,* involving the left adrenal gland and extending to a perirenal space and the upper pole of the kidney. **c** Pulmonary metastases demonstrating differing growth patterns depending on the different primary tumor; expansile on the right, from a *hepatic cell carcinoma,* and infiltrating and irregularly contoured on the left, from a *mammary carcinoma.* The different origin of the two metastases was confirmed at autopsy

mandates rigorous respect for the timing of data acquisition in relation to the contrast bolus administration.

Modern helical CT technology, due to the ever improving speed of data acquisition, allows now sophisticated chronologic tailoring of the examination in order to maximize clinical information in any particular anatomic district in relation to the clinical issue to be addressed.

As previously underlined, the metastatization process follows complex rules, depending on the intrinsic characteristic of the primary neoplasm and, to a lesser extent, upon loco-regional and host factors. Thus, knowledge of the specific patterns of metastatic colonization and of their usual and less usual structural features

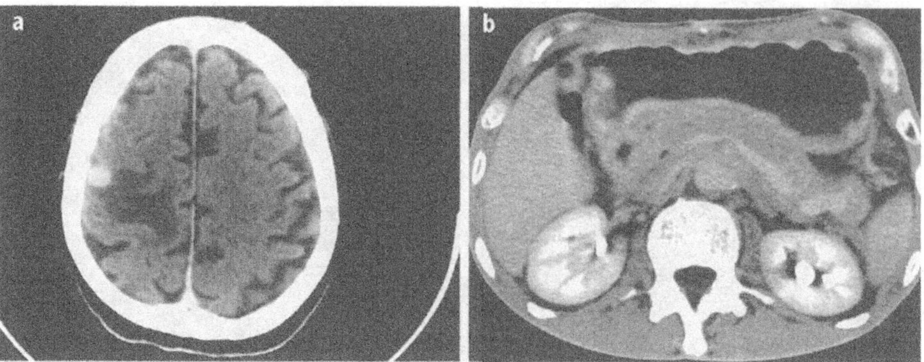

Fig. 6. a Cerebral metastasis from a *pulmonary adenocarcinoma*, surrounded by gross perilesional edema. **b** Diffuse lymphangitic infiltration of the pancreatic parenchyma, secondary to a *sigmoid adenocarcinoma*, with marked secondary desmoplastic reaction

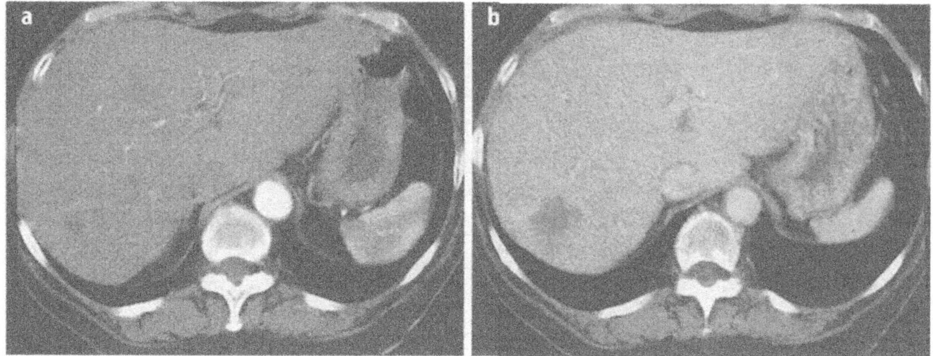

Fig. 7. Hepatic metastasis from a *colon carcinoma* **a** in arterial and **b** portal venous phase

(calcification, pseudocystic degeneration, hemorrhage, hypervascularization, etc.) represents the indispensable requirement for a correct radiologic approach, both at staging and during follow-up.

▪ Calcified Metastases

The pathogenetic process of calcification within a metastatic lesion is complex and not yet entirely clarified in all of its aspects [5,6]. Calcium salts deposition within a metastatic deposit appears to indeed have a multifactorial genesis, although the histologic type of the primary tumor seems to be the single most important factor. Different histologic types display different calcification patterns [26].

Two basic types of calcification process are commonly recognized: The first type is typical of those histotypes in which the calcification occurs primarily intralesionally, as an inherent and proprietary characteristic of the neoplastic cell [23]. It is the so-called Orthoplastic calcification, typically seen in metastases from osteo-

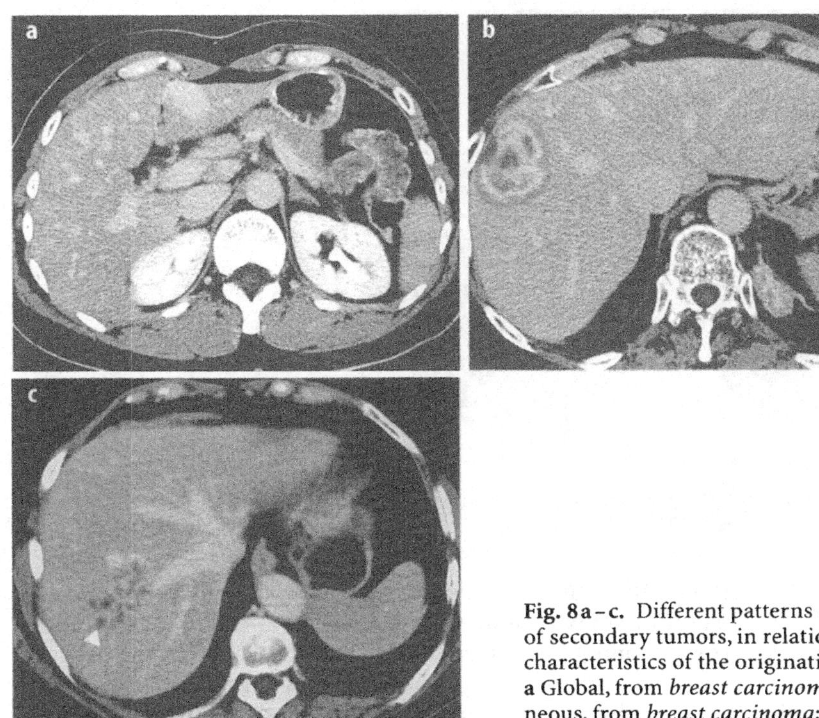

Fig. 8a–c. Different patterns of enhancement of secondary tumors, in relation to the vascular characteristics of the originating primaries. **a** Global, from *breast carcinoma*; **b** heterogeneous, from *breast carcinoma*; **c** peripheral ring enhancement (*arrowhead*) from *bronchogenic carcinoma*

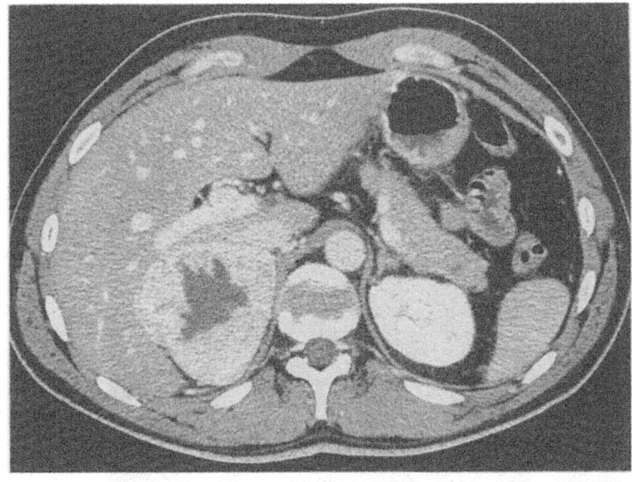

Fig. 9. Hypervascular metastasis to the right adrenal gland, secondary to an *anaplastic small cell carcinoid of the lung*, with gross central necrotic involution

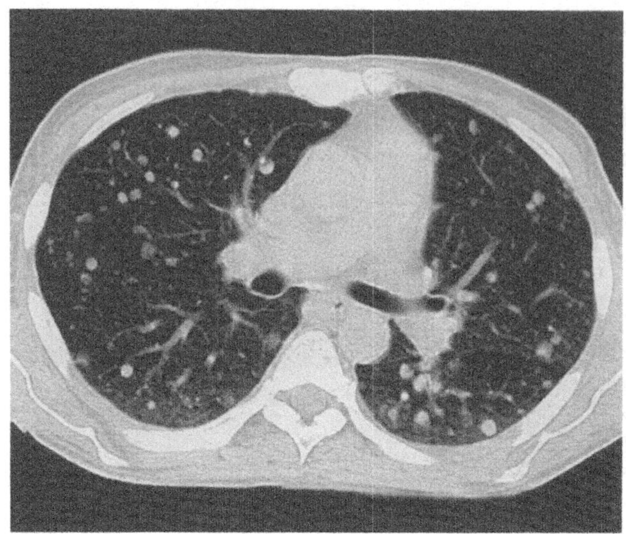

Fig. 10. Massive hematogenous metastatization to the lungs, secondary to a *clear cell renal carcinoma*

sarcoma (Fig. 12). This results from an actual, albeit atypical, ossifying process occurring within the osteoid matrix produced by the tumoral cells [26, 27]. These premises explain the grossly homogeneous and compact appearance of the calcium depositions encompassing the vast majority of the tumoral volume [26, 28].

Pathogenetically similar is the process that ultimately leads to the Metaplastic calcification of chondrosarcomas, in which the amorphous structure of the metastasis is due to the transformation of the neoplastic cartilaginous tissue toward bony tissue, through a pathway which is analogous to that of enchondral ossification (Fig. 13) [23].

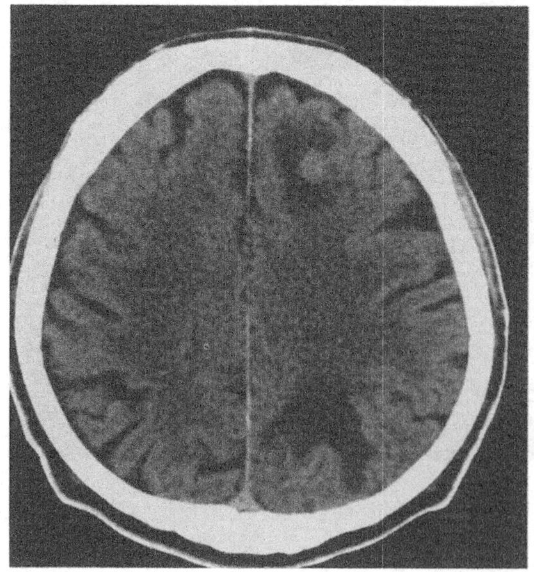

Fig. 11. Hyperdense cerebral metastasis with perilesional edema, from *small cell lung cancer*

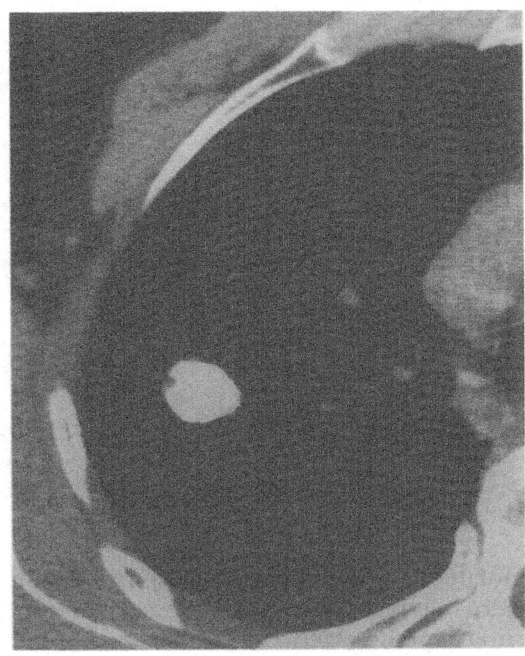

Fig. 12. Pulmonary metastasis with marked homogeneous calcification, of the orthoplastic type, secondary to a *femoral osteosarcoma*

The second mechanism, certainly more common and seen in many epithelial neoplasms, is the Dystrophic calcification [6, 29]. This is essentially thought to represent a stromal reaction to a vascular injury, such as ischemia, necrosis, and/or hemorrhage. All of these processes probably alter the microenvironmental conditions, particularly the acidity of the medium, therefore triggering calcium deposition [29]. Ischemia is considered the most important initiating factor. The

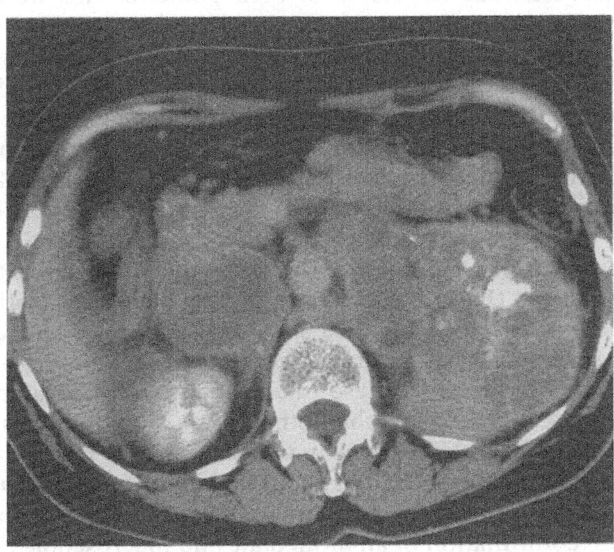

Fig. 13. Metastasis to the left kidney, with metaplastic calcification, secondary to a *chondrosarcoma of the orbit.* Note the concurrent neoplastic thrombosis of the left renal vein and inferior vena cava

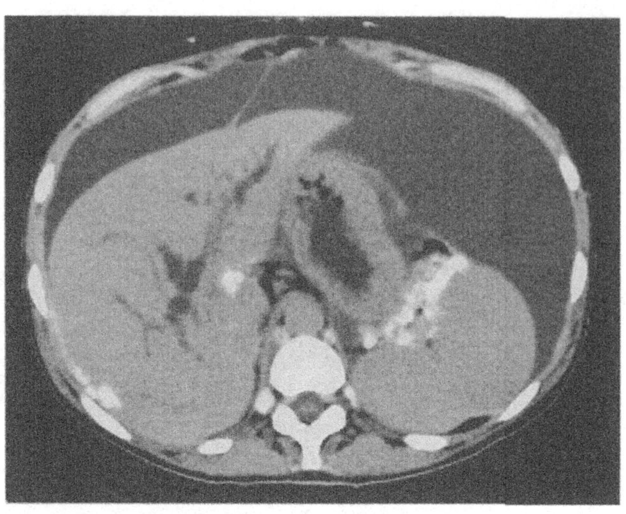

Fig. 14. Peritoneal metastases with psammomatous calcifications, from a *papillary cystadenocarcinoma of the ovary*

amorphous component of calcium deposits is more often central in location, where hypoxia and necrosis are more prominent. This pattern seems to confirm the primary pathogenetic role of ischemia [30].

A particular variety of dystrophic calcification, the Psammomatous type, is characteristic of papillary epithelial neoplasms of the ovary and thyroid, and is also described in mesotheliomas and bronchiolo-alveolar carcinomas (Fig. 14). All of these tumors are associated with pathologic evidence of "psammoma bodies," which are described as concentrically arranged calcium conglomerates, in the form of needle-shaped crystals and with ultrastructural and X-ray refractive features resembling those of hydroxyapatite [30]. The papillary structures typical of these malignancies are believed to offer a favorable anatomic background for ischemic necrosis, due to torsion of their pedicles. This would be followed by autophagic phenomena of the superficial cellular layer and by ischemic necrosis of the entire papilla with release of lipidic vesicles which would act as an organic substrate for the precipitation of calcium salts [30]. The cytoplasmic microfilaments, which abound in most papillary tumors, are also believed to represent an additional favoring factor, maybe acting as a skeleton for the psammoma body. The coalescence of these microscopic structures results in the creation of a calcification macroscopically recognized both in the primary and the secondary neoplasm [30].

Another dystrophic variant, the Mucoid-type calcification, occurs in mucin-secreting carcinomas of the gastrointestinal tract, the breast, the ovary, and the pancreas (Fig. 15). Debris originating from degradation of glycoprotein and mucopolysaccharides secreted by neoplastic cells and associated with necrosis and hemorrhage are the probable causes of calcium deposits [6, 28].

Although all of these calcifications occur in a spontaneous fashion, they may also be secondary to chemotherapy or radiation. This holds true particularly for the dystrophic calcifications in which treatment may enhance tissue-regressive phenomena, with further amorphous precipitation of calcium [26]. This peculiar response to therapy is particularly apparent in metastases from ovarian carcinomas, in which the combination of an immediate and macroscopic tissue response to specific anti-

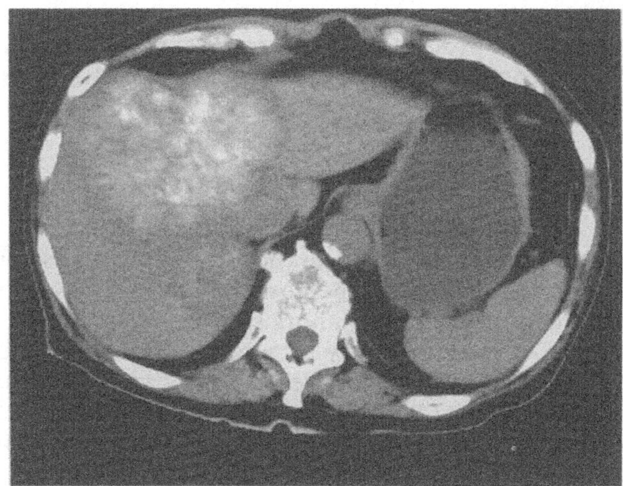

Fig. 15. Large metastatic deposit in the liver, with gross mucoid-type calcifications, secondary to a *mucinous adenocarcinoma of the colon*

tumoral therapy and the inherent characteristics of this often mucinous tumor leads to cases of massive intratumoral calcifications (Fig. 16). Such events may thus represent a clue to the biological quiescence of the lesion, with favorable clinical implications for the patient.

The reported incidence of calcified metastases in the literature is remarkably variable (2–27%), probably because of different histologies and organs primarily involved. Gastrointestinal and ovarian adenocarcinomas, osteosarcomas, and papillary carcinomas of the thyroid are the most frequently responsible histologic types, with liver, lung, lymph nodes, and peritoneum being the most frequently affected sites [26]. The morphologic appearance of the calcification itself may be starry, poppy seeds, ring-like, granular, or massively coarse, and is often associated with a peripheral hypodense component, especially during the active deposition of calcium [26].

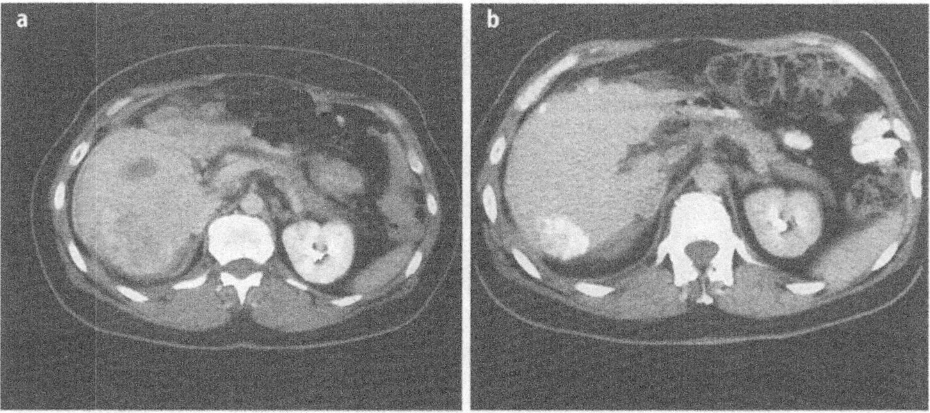

Fig. 16a,b. Progressive deposition of calcium salts within the substance of hepatic metastases from an *ovarian carcinoma*, after completion of chemotherapy (**b**)

The most common non-neoplastic calcified diseases include parasitic and granulomatous processes. These entities, along with primary benign or malignant tumors, compose the differential diagnostic list, which changes according to the organ in consideration.

■ Pseudocystic Metastases

The pseudocystic appearance of metastases is caused, just as in the primary neoplasms, by extensive necrosis and myxoid degeneration. Necrosis is particularly prominent in primary tumors such as breast cancer, sarcomas, and colon cancer, because of their tendency to outgrow their blood supply due to their tumultuous growth, or may be alternatively secondary to efficacious radiation or chemotherapy treatment (Fig. 17) [31]. The ensuing necrotic liquefaction is not limited to the central portion, as in most lesions of critical size, but involves the whole lesion (Fig. 18) [23].

The CT appearance is that of masses with homogeneously hypodense content (HU readings of 0–20), with a thick and seldom irregular wall, which displays some contrast enhancement after intravenous contrast administration. Thin septa and intracavitary debris are not an unusual finding [23].

Liver, brain, peritoneum, ovary, and lymph nodes are the sites most frequently involved, although this aspect can potentially be found in any organ.

■ Cavitation of Metastases

Cavitation is a typical complication of pulmonary secondary tumors (Fig. 10). A few cases have also been described in the small bowel [32, 33]. Although the exact modality of occurrence has not yet been completely demonstrated, this process is believed to be secondary to a valve mechanism which allows emptying of massively

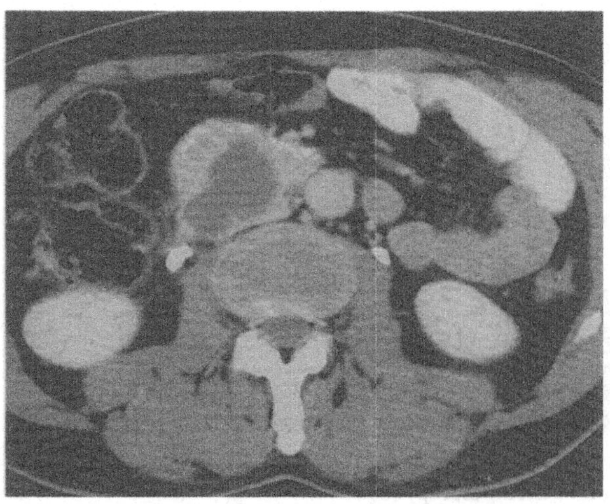

Fig. 17. Pseudocystic metastases to retroperitoneal lymph nodes, from an *embryonal carcinoma of the testis,* after completion of chemotherapy

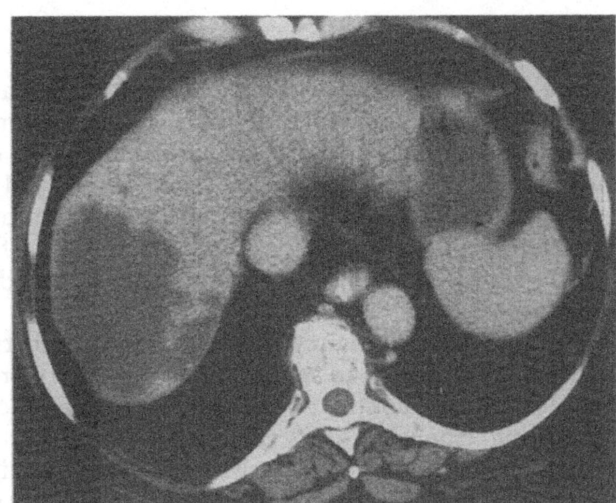

Fig. 18. Pseudeocystic metatasis to the liver, from a *colon carcinoma*, characterized by massive central necrotic colliquation

necrotic lesions into the bronchial tree after neoplastic infiltration of structures directly communicating with the airway. If the lesion is in a subpleural location, a pneumothorax may alternatively occur [34, 35].

The incidence of cavitated lesions among all pulmonary secondary tumors is approximately 4 %; of these, 70 % occur in squamous cell carcinomas, most frequently originating in the head, neck, and female genital system [32, 36]. Much more rarely, metastases from colon cancer and soft tissue sarcomas, as well as lesions regressing after chemotherapy, may exhibit this peculiar appearance [37].

The walls in these tumors are variably thick and generally very irregular, but they may sometimes be as thin as those seen in coccidioidomycosis (Fig. 19) [38]. Solitary forms must be differentiated from a primary lung cancer or infectious cavitating diseases (tuberculosis, mycosis, etc.) [39].

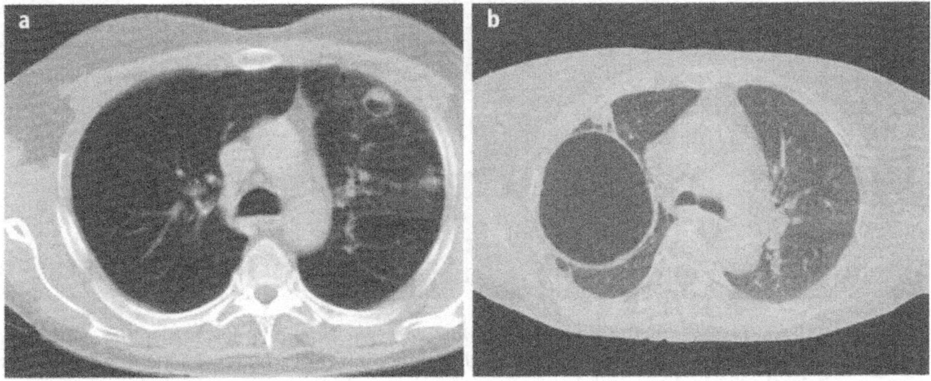

Fig. 19. Cavitary pulmonary metastases from **a** a *squamous cell carcinoma of the maxillary sinus* and **b** a *uterine sarcoma*

■ Cystic Metastases

The cystic appearance of a metastasis is generally a secondary expression of a primary malignancy in which the specific cellular differentiation determines, ab initio, a predominately cystic structure, not due to necrotic events [23, 40]. Tumors such as pancreatic macrocystic carcinomas and ovarian cystadenocarcinomas exhibit extensive serous or mucinous production, according to the physiologic differentiation of the primary tumor. The density of the cystic content is therefore strictly fluid (−5/+20 HU) in serous tumors or slightly higher (20/30 HU) in mucinous tumors.

The signs of malignancy within a cystic lesion are represented by focal or diffuse thickenings of walls and septa (Fig. 11), papillary projections, solid nodules, irregular calcifications, contrast enhancement of the solid component, and extracapsular infiltrating extension into the surrounding tissues (Fig. 20) [23]. In addition, knowledge of the patient's positive history for malignancy as well as knowledge of the type of primary tumor involved may allow a specific characterization of the lesion; otherwise, in the presence of an inconclusive history, differential diagnosis versus complex-appearing cystic lesions of the liver, kidney, and ovary (hydatid disease, other primary cystic tumors) may be virtually impossible.

■ Hemorrhagic Metastases

Metastases tend to reproduce the vascular characteristics of the primary neoplasm; thus, lesions secondary to a hypervascular primary (hypernephroma, pheochromocytoma, malignant Apudomas, carcinoids, melanomas, leiomyosarcomas, thyroid carcinomas, granulose cell tumors, chorioncarcinomas, hemangiosarcomas, malignant schwannomas) are accordingly hypervascular and exhibit tendency toward hemorrhage [6, 23, 41]. However, hemorrhagic phenomena have also been

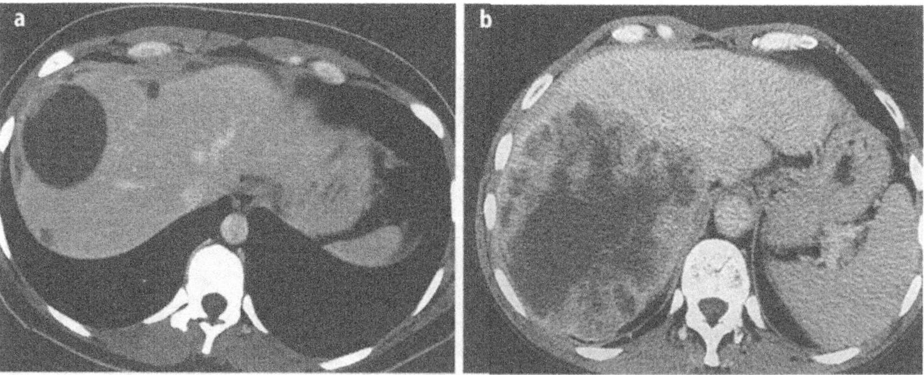

Fig. 20. a Cystic metastasis to the liver from a *mucoid cystic adenocarcinoma of the gallbladder*, containing fluid and a large papillary solid mural nodule on its anterolateral aspect. **b** Large metastatic deposit in the right hepatic lobe, with extensive cystic features, secondary to a *mucinous macrocystic adenocarcinoma of the pancreas*. The lesion demonstrates thick walls and intralesional septa

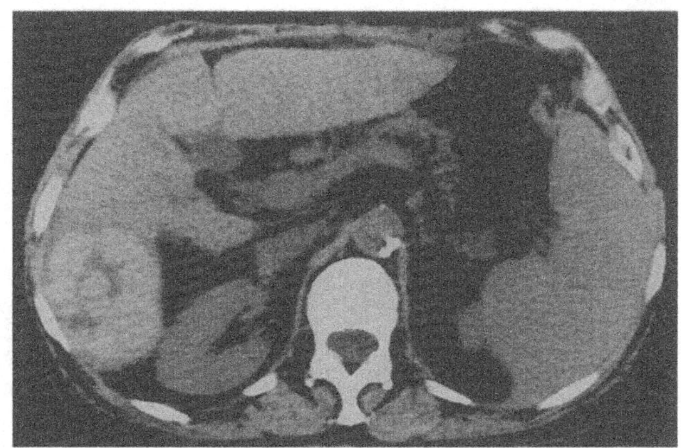

Fig. 21. Large metastatic deposit to the liver, from a melanoma, which at baseline demonstrates the classical heterogeneous hyperdensity of an acute hemorrhagic complication

described within hypovascular metastases (breast and colon carcinoma), and occasionally in patients undergoing anticoagulant therapies. The clinical appearance may be severe, as is sometimes seen in hemorrhagic metastases of the liver which may present with acute abdominal symptoms, hemoperitoneum, and shock.

The appearance of hemorrhagic lesions, despite the peculiarities due to the affected organ (liver, kidney, adrenal, brain, and bowel are the most frequent locations), basically depends on the stage and age of the hemorrhage [42, 43]. In the acute phase an intralesional heterogeneous hyperdensity (Fig. 21) is present at baseline scanning [43]. When the lesion is superficially located in relation to the surface of the organ, extension of the hemorrhage within the subcapsular and extracapsular spaces is possible, with frank perivisceral blood collections. The structural evolution of hemorrhagic lesions is in substance the one of blood catabolism, with liquefaction of the clot and a progression toward hypodensity which may border that of water [43, 44]. In these older stages, differentiation between a cyst and an old hemorrhage may become arduous [45]. In the majority of these cases, focal or diffuse wall thickenings, septa, intralesional debris or fluid–fluid levels (Fig. 22), HU values even slightly above the ones of cysts, coupled with a specific history, may all lead toward a correct diagnosis. An additional clue may be offered by the careful analysis of the intralesional attenuation values before and after contrast medium administration, which may demonstrate slight contrast enhancement in chronic hemorrhagic metastases [23].

■ Lipoid Metastases

Lipoid metastases are metastatic deposits from primary malignancies with extensive representation of lipomatous tissue, such as liposarcoma, immature teratomas, and sarcomas with mixed cellularity and/or lipidic component. The CT ability to characterize lesions, or portions of lesions, as lipoid (HU values of −150/−25) rests on the relatively homogeneous representation of discrete foci of lipoid tissue in the volume of interest. However, such event is rare. For example, areas of negative HU values are mostly found within well-differentiated liposarcomas, which in fact are less likely to metastatize than other subtypes; in the myxoid variant, fluid

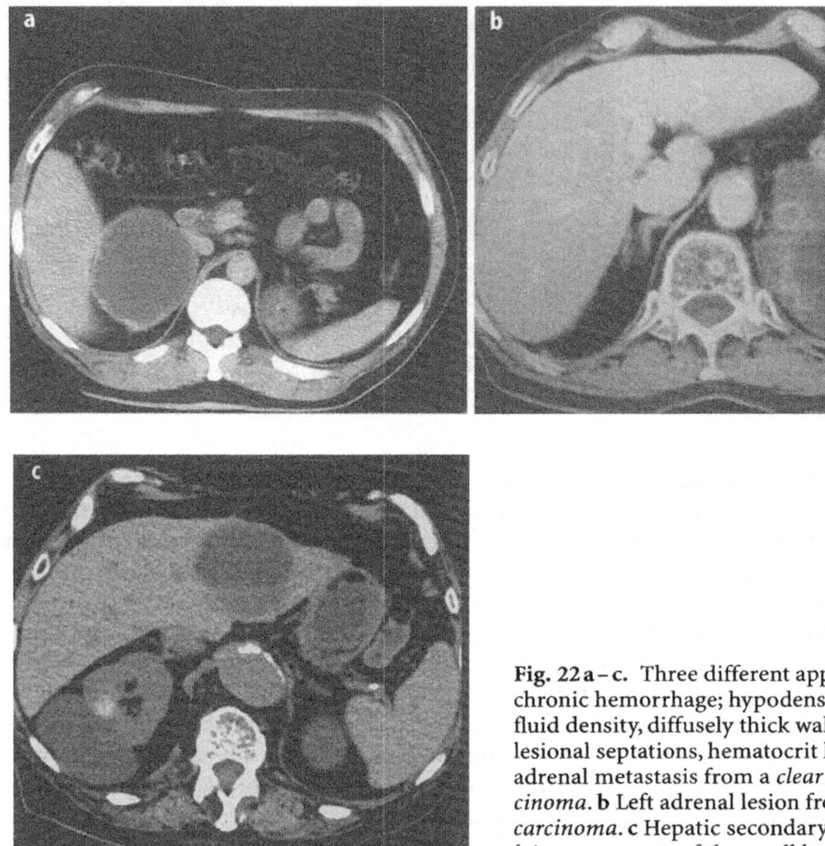

Fig. 22a–c. Three different appearances of chronic hemorrhage; hypodensity with frank fluid density, diffusely thick walls with endo-lesional septations, hematocrit level. **a** Right adrenal metastasis from a *clear cell renal carcinoma*. **b** Left adrenal lesion from a *colonic carcinoma*. **c** Hepatic secondary tumor from a *leiomyosarcoma of the small bowel*

or fluid-like densitometric values prevail, due to averaging of the lipidic and solid or mucinous tumoral components; highly undifferentiated forms, such as the pleomorphic or round-cell variants, with their marked cellularity, have a strictly solid appearance. Chemotherapy, by causing intralesional necrosis, may also obliterate adipose densities.

Malignant teratomas rarely metastasize, and their secondary lesions occasionally display calcified areas. In such lesions CT may be extremely helpful, identifying "retroconversion" to mature elements, without evolutionary potentials, by demonstrating better defined margins, increase in size and number of calcifications, and better demarcation of the adipose component (Fig. 23) [46]. Lung, liver, and peritoneum are the most frequent organs of localization of lipoid metastases.

■ Infected Metastases

The superimposition of infectious processes on a neoplastic lesion is not a very common event in the evolution of a metastasis. Immune deficiencies (leukemia,

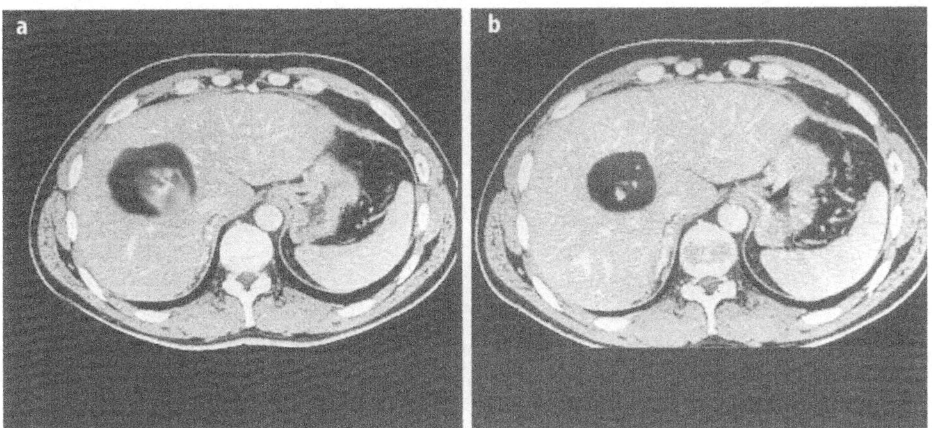

Fig. 23. a Hepatic metastasis from an immature ovarian teratoma, with frankly adipose areas.
b After chemotherapy, the lesion is smaller, with interval decrease of the solid component and
marked increase in the extent of calcification phenomena

AIDS, bone marrow transplant) or massively necrotic lesions (chemoembolization)
are the most frequent clinical situations in which infectious complications take
place [23].

In addition to a more or less suggestive clinical picture, which may be as
simple as a low-grade fever, the CT appearance is abscess-like, with evidence of
a fluid lesion demarcated by a more or less thick and irregularly enhancing border
and with occasional enhancing septa [47]. Where gas-producing agents are
involved, the detection of gas bubbles or air–fluid levels is extremely helpful
(Fig. 24) [20].

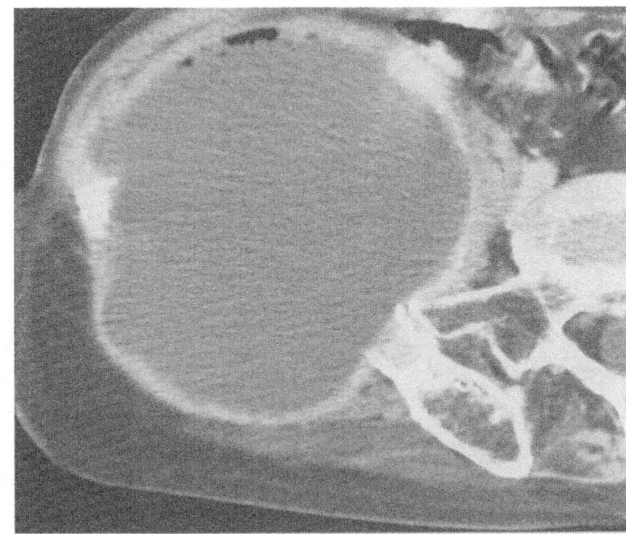

Fig. 24. Voluminous soft
tissue mass of the right ilium,
with extensive necrosis, from
a papillary carcinoma of the
thyroid, demonstrating peripheral ring enhancement
and multiple intralesional gas
bubbles. This appearance was
due to superinfection from
anaerobic microorganisms

CHAPTER 4

Anatomical Sites of Metastatic Colonization

■ Classical Targets

Cerebrum

The brain is one of the most important targets of metastatic tumoral involvement, with frequency ranging from 4 to 37% [20, 25, 48]. Metastases represent the most frequent neoplastic pathology of the central nervous system, constituting approximately 20% of all clinically evident tumors. Their incidence is particularly high between the fourth and seventh decade, without gender preference [20, 25, 49].

Whereas their origin is most often hematogenous, cerebral metastases are occasionally secondary to spread by contiguity from primary lesions of the dura or skull base [7]. The supratentorial district is most frequently affected (80% of cases) [50]. The exception is represented by metastases from renal cell carcinomas, which exhibit a surprising affinity for the infratentorial district [7].

Intra-axial lesions appear to be the most frequent ones. Bronchogenic carcinomas, especially of the small cell and anaplastic types, are the most common originating primary tumor, followed by breast, renal, gastrointestinal cancers, and melanomas. They are generally multiple (60–85% of cases), although there is a statistically significant portion of solitary lesions, particularly in relation to melanomas as well as, bronchogenic and breast carcinomas [20].

The gray–white matter junction typically represents the site of initial neoplastic implantation, probably because of the marked narrowing of the arterioles at this level. Vasogenic peritumoral edema, secondary to altered vascular permeability, involves predominantly the white matter, rarely the cortex (probably due to its lack of interstitium) [24, 48], and does not cross the corpus callosum. Its extent is only partially related to the dimension of the tumor deposit. The rare intraventricular metastases are more often found in the lateral ventricles [51].

On non-enhanced CT images the majority of cerebral metastases appear isodense with the surrounding parenchyma [25]. Those lesions secondary to tumors with a high nucleus/cytoplasm ratio, such as small cell lung cancer, or with secretory ability, such as mucoid gastrointestinal carcinomas, often appear hyperdense (Fig. 4) [50]. A recent report described a markedly hyperdense metastatic deposit from an adenocarcinoma, in which pathology described coagulative necrosis with a high protein content, without hemorrhagic or calcified components [52]. Hemorrhagic complications with their classic hyperdense appearance in the acute stage are typical of renal and breast carcinomas, chorioncarcinomas, and melanomas [44]. Cystic or calcified lesions have been described in 1–6.6% of cases in the literature

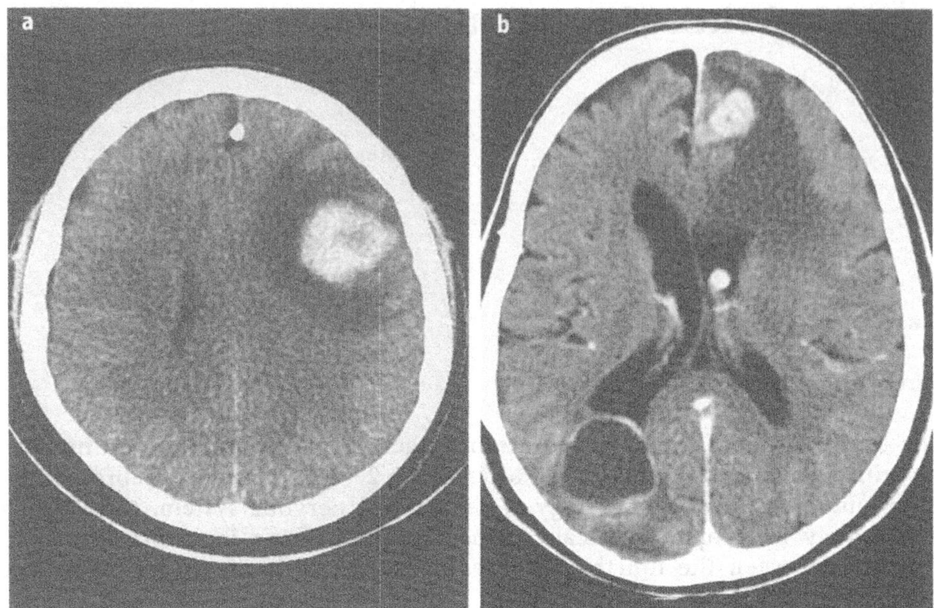

Fig. 25. Hemorrhagic metastases to the brain from **a** *melanoma* and **b** *parathyroid carcinoma*

and are mostly secondary to bronchogenic, mammary, and ovarian carcinomas, and to osteosarcomas (Fig. 25) [49–50].

The majority of lesions exhibit marked contrast enhancement secondary to alterations in the blood-brain barrier. The enhancing pattern may be solid nodular, ring-like, due to extensive central necrosis, or inhomogenous with irregular contours (Fig. 26) [50]. The administration of double-dose intravenous contrast and delayed imaging markedly increases the sensitivity of contrast-enhanced CT.

Abscesses, multifocal gliomas and meningiomas, lymphomatous masses, and tubercular or parasitic lesions all represent primary differential diagnostic considerations in the presence of multiple metastases [49]. Several primary tumors, astrocytomas, and others must instead be considered in the presence of a solitary mass [49]. If the process is located in the posterior fossa, the hemangioblastoma and lymphoma are the main differential diagnostic possibilities.

Extra-axial lesions are not a rare occurrence; approximately 18% of patients with intracranial metastases demonstrate dural localizations as the only site of neoplastic colonization. These are more often secondary to neuroblastomas, or breast and prostate carcinomas (Fig. 27) [48]. The epidural locations, generally secondary to hematogenous diffusion through the epidural venous plexus, are due mostly to an adjacent bone metastasis from breast, lung, prostate, or thyroid carcinomas [7]. Venous thrombosis is also a possible complication of the tumoral invasion of the dural sinuses or, more rarely, of venous compression and stasis. Leptomeningeal carcinomatosis, secondary to involvement of the subarachnoid space and of skull base structures, is generally the expression of metastatic diffusion from gastric, pulmonary, breast, and ovarian carcinomas, as well as melanomas and selected primary cerebral tumors [1, 7]. Diffuse thickening of the skull base lepto-

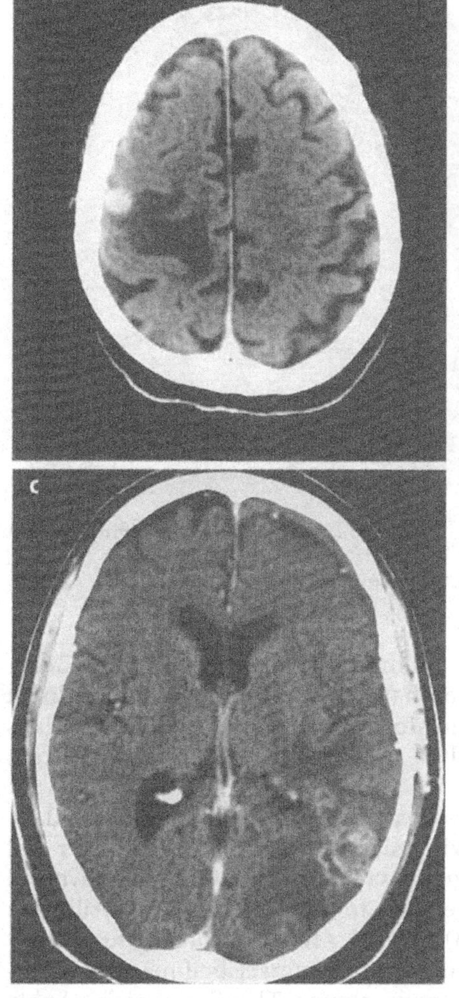
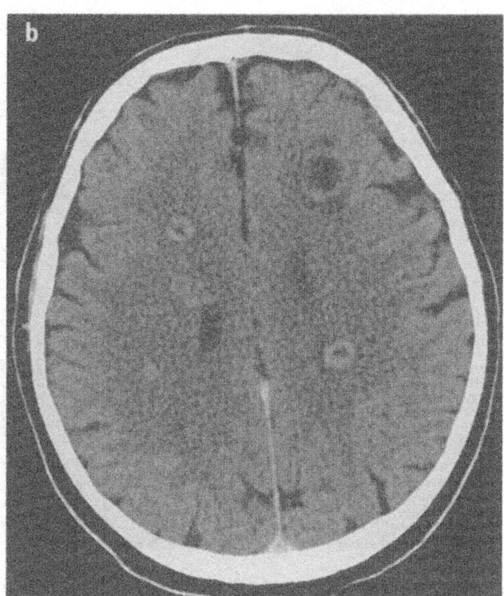

Fig. 26. Cerebral metastases, from *bronchogenic carcinoma*, with marked contrast enhancement, appearing as **a** solid nodule, **b** ring-enhancing nodule and **c** as heterogeneous density in an irregularly contoured lesion

meningeal lining is frequently associated with metastatic infiltrates extending along the perivascular spaces and into the cerebral parenchyma, with a secondary fibroblastic reaction of the meninges themselves [53].

Lung

The lung is the most frequent organ of metastatic involvement, with disease present in 20–54% of patients deceased from extrathoracic neoplastic disease [20]. From autopsy studies breast, uterus, kidney, and head and neck cancers are the primary tumors that most frequently metastasize to the lungs [20, 38]. Chorioncarcinomas, osteosarcomas, melanomas, Ewing's sarcomas, melanomas, and thyroid carcinomas follow in order of frequency [7, 54].

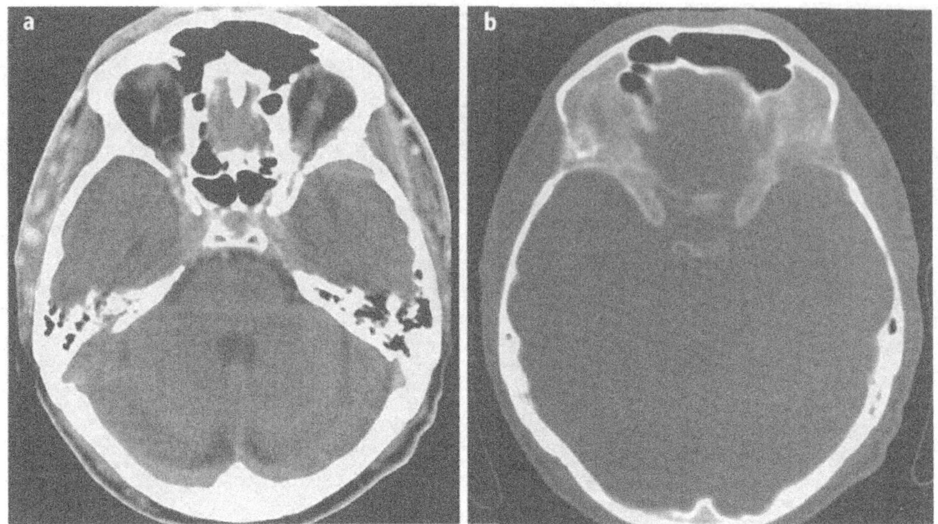

Fig. 27 a, b. Secondary osteomeningeal localization from a *breast carcinoma*, involving the left pterion. **a** There is thickening of the meninges at the level of the anterior pole of the left temporal lobe, with **b** ballooning and demineralization of the lateral wall of the orbit

From the pathogenetic point of view, pulmonary localization may occur through five different pathways: arterial, lymphatic, pleural, airborne, and direct invasion. Hematogenous diffusion is by far the most frequent, and tumors of organs the venous drainage of which directly involves the lung are the most significant primary causes [7].

The most frequent appearance of pulmonary metastases is characterized by bilateral multiple nodules of markedly varying size [38, 54]. The lung bases and the subpleural peripheral portions of parenchyma are most frequently involved (82–92% according to autopsy studies), in relation to the preferential distribution of the pulmonary arterial blood flow (Fig. 28) [20, 38]. Always according to autopsy studies, 30% of the nodules exhibit well-defined and circumscribed margins, without gross signs of invasion of the surrounding parenchyma. This finding is probably related to the hematogenous origin of these lesions, with a cellular proliferation which takes place entirely within the perivascular interstitium [12]. The neoplastic proliferation may subsequently extend along the interstitial spaces and/or into the adjacent alveolar spaces, destroying the parenchyma and therefore causing irregular borders (Fig. 29) [55]. Subpleural locations, "plaque-like" appearance, and stellate contours are additional, not unusual, morphologic features [12]. A typical example is hepatocellular carcinoma, the expansile growth of which causes well-defined and regular margins. On the other hand, metastatic adenocarcinomas, epidermoid carcinomas, and metastases after chemotherapy more often exhibit ill-defined and variably smooth contours [55].

Such variability in appearance often causes differential diagnostic dilemmas, which are occasionally amenable only to histopathologic analysis. Benign lesions, such as hamartomas or granulomas, may not be differentiated from metastases with well-defined borders [12]. On the other hand, an ill-contoured metastasis may not

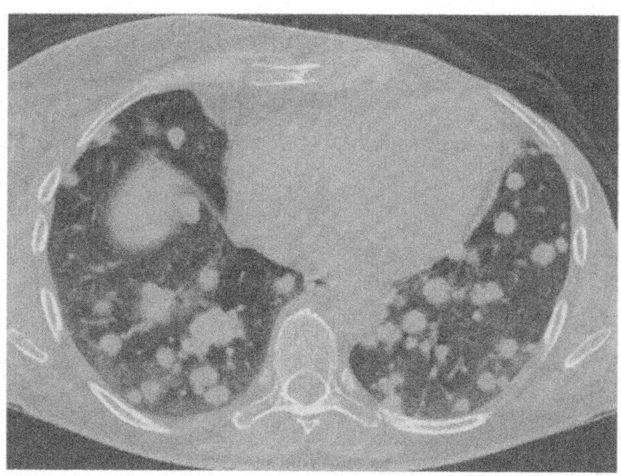

Fig. 28. Massive bilateral pulmonary metastatization from *breast carcinoma*

be discriminated by a primary pulmonary tumor. A typical feature, easily documented by CT, is the direct connection between a tumoral deposit and a pulmonary vessel. Such a finding, also documented at angiography, allows reliable assessment of the hematogenous origin of the lesion. The presence of a possible perinodular hypodensity may reflect a reduced blood perfusion secondary to neoplastic obstruction of the pulmonary arterial branch [12]. Although it is not always possible to define a parallel between the macroscopic appearance of metastases and their causative primary tumor [56, 57], there are histologic types which are more

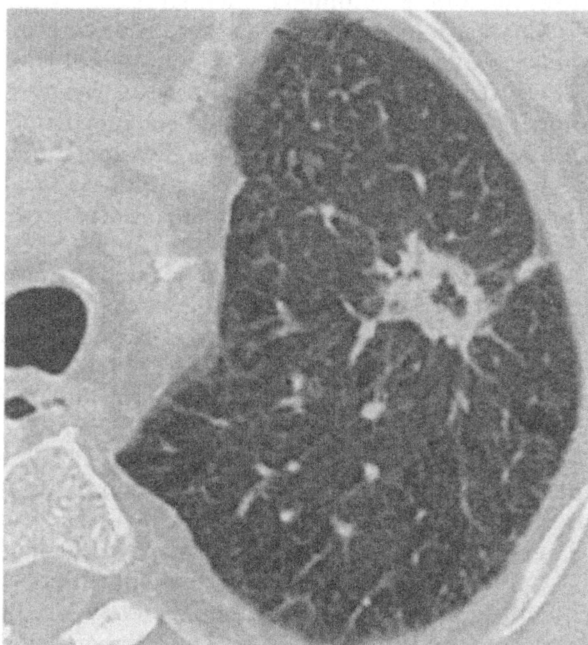

Fig. 29. Pulmonary secondary melanoma, characterized by irregular and stellate contour, which is the expression of the neoplastic growth along the interstitium and the adjacent alveolar spaces, causing destruction of the alveolar parenchyma

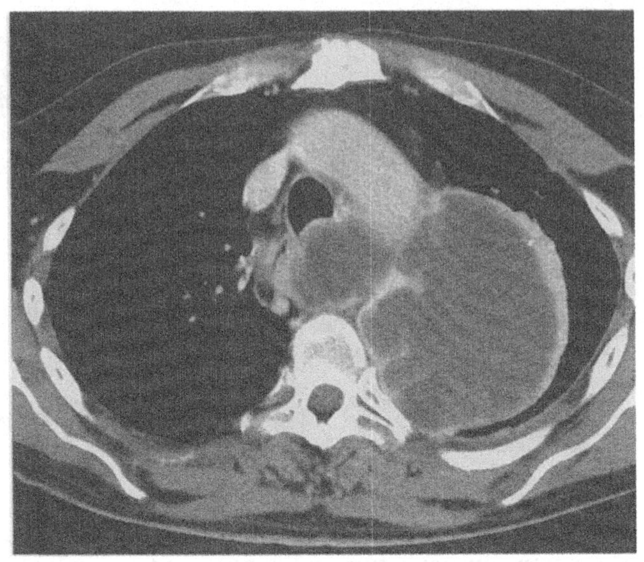

Fig. 30. Pseudocystic metastasis of the lung, with irregular thick walls, secondary to a *malignant fibrous histiocytoma of the retroperitoneum*, currently undergoing chemotherapy. There is a virtually complete necrotic degeneration with irregular intralesional septa

frequently associated with selected morphologic features. For example, a miliary diffusion is often seen in metastatic diffusion from medullary carcinomas of the thyroid, whereas large multiple nodules are frequently detected in patients with renal cell carcinomas, chorioncarcinomas, melanomas, seminomas, and sarcomas (Fig. 28) [55].

The metastatic nodules, often homogeneous in density if small, tend to display central necrotic phenomena when large [56], with subtotal colliquation typically seen in large lesions after chemotherapy or with selected tumors such as sarcomas or breast and colon carcinomas (Fig. 30) [23, 27].

The growth dynamics of metastases varies widely depending on the primary tumors. They may display an indolent growth of metastatic thyroid or salivary adenoid-cystic carcinomas, with a doubling time of several months. They may display highly aggressive growth patterns, as in osteosarcomas, melanomas, and germ cell tumors of the testes, the metastases of which may double in diameter in 1–2 weeks [12].

The solitary lesion is a less frequent but much more challenging diagnostic scenario. It is presently widely believed that a second primary tumor, especially in the metachronous phase, is a statistically more significant occurrence (60%) than a solitary delayed metastatic deposit (24%) [55]. It is useful to remember in this context that patients with epitheliomas of the head and neck region, pulmonary, mammary, gastric, or prostate carcinomas are more likely to develop a second primary tumor in the lung rather that exhibit a solitary metastatic pulmonary deposit. The latter finding, in contrast, is more probable in patients with melanomas, sarcomas, or colon carcinomas which may give rise to solitary metastases [55].

There are multiple factors which may influence the morphologic appearance of a pulmonary metastasis and therefore tissue characterization. Hemorrhage, frequently seen in metastases from hemangiosarcomas or chorioncarcinomas, may determine variations mostly at the periphery of the lesion [12, 55, 56] where it

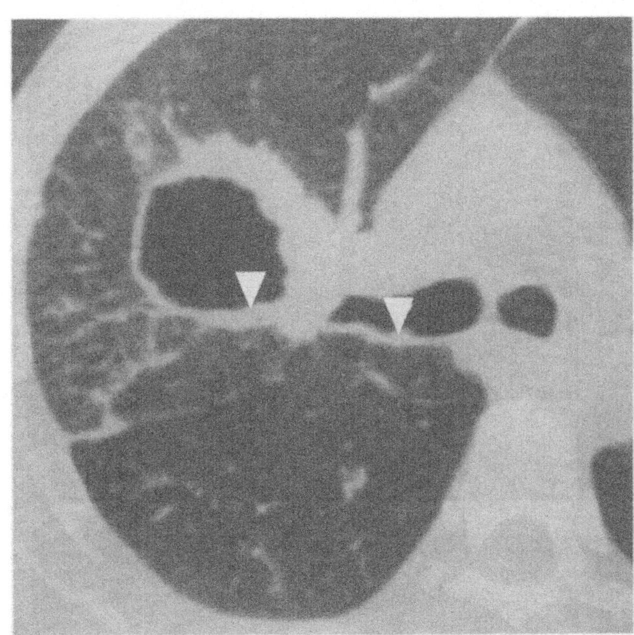

Fig. 31. Cavitated metastasis of the lung from a *uterine leiomyosarcoma*. Computed tomography accurately depicts the marked and irregular thickening of the wall, the draining bronchus, and the intralesional and endobronchial neoplastic papillae (*arrowheads*)

may cause a relatively specific ground-glass appearance or an ill-defined irregular contour, the latter also present in active tubercular lesions [58], in aspergillosis [59], or after a biopsy [60]. Abscesses or lymphomatous localizations in immuno-compromised patients may analogously cause alterations of a lesion's contour due to deposition of fibrin, inflammatory response, or perilesional edema [56,61]. Cavitary lesions account for approximately 4–6% of pulmonary metastases and are secondary to squamous cell carcinomas in 70% of cases [32]. Neoplasms of the head and neck and, in women, of the genital system are the most frequent originating primary tumors [36], followed by colon carcinomas and sarcomas [55]. The CT appearance of cavitary metastases is variable: Their walls are often thick and irregular, although sometimes very thin, in all similar to the coccidioidomycosis processes (Figs. 19, 31) [55].

Very infrequent are metastases with a lipoid component, secondary to liposarcomas or immature teratomas (Fig. 32), and with calcifications. It is useful to remember that, although the presence of calcium within a pulmonary lesion is almost universally accepted as a sign of benignity (hamartoma, granuloma), calcified metastases have nevertheless been described, especially in relation to selected histologic types [28]. It is the case of metastases from osteosarcomas (Fig. 12) and chondrosarcomas, characterized by a dominant calcified matrix, compact in appearance and predominantly eccentric in location. Metastases from mucin-secreting adenocarcinomas of the breast or gastrointestinal system, as well as papillary tumors of the ovary or thyroid, may also be characterized by dusty or punctate calcifications (Fig. 33), especially after chemotherapy treatment (Fig. 3) [28]. Extremely rare, on the other hand, is the occurrence of calcification within primary lung tumors, especially adenocarcinomas, carcinoids, or hemangiopericytomas [55].

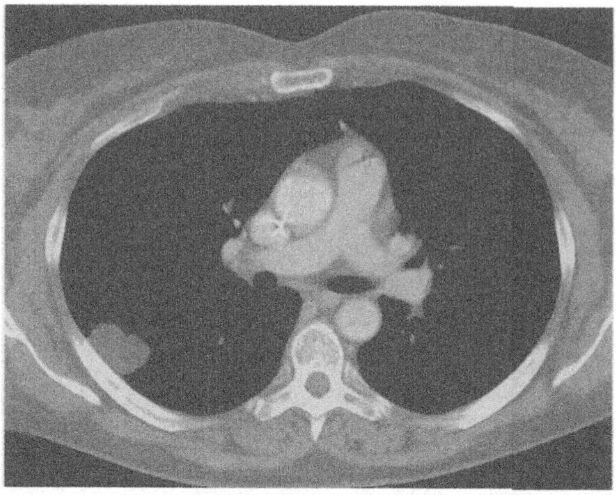

Fig. 32. Pulmonary metastasis with homogeneous fatty density, secondary to a *retroperitoneal myxoid liposarcoma*

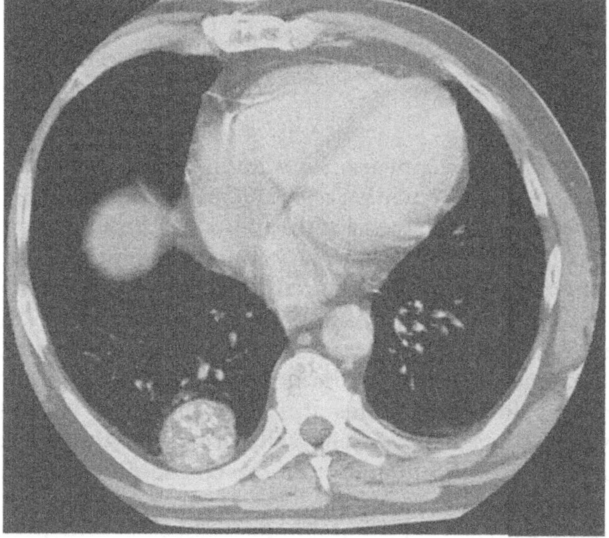

Fig. 33. Pulmonary metastasis from a *mucoid adenocarcinoma of the colon*, exhibiting multiple punctate calcifications

Endobronchial metastases are also rare. They are most often secondary to cancers of the kidney, colon, breast, and pancreas (Fig. 34) [62]. Possible mechanisms include lymphatic or hematogenous diffusion, direct spread from contiguous parenchymal, mediastinal, or nodal lesions, or, less likely, air-borne diffusion [55]. The incidence of macroscopic endobronchial repetitions varies in the literature from 1.1 to 18%. Much more frequently (70%) they are detected at microscopic examination [12]. Their radiologic detection is rare and is generally suspected by underlying specific symptoms, such as cough, dyspnea, and hemoptysis, indicating an advanced stage of the disease [55]. Oligohemia is the main indirect radiographic sign, in association with atelectasis or post-obstructive pneumonitis [12].

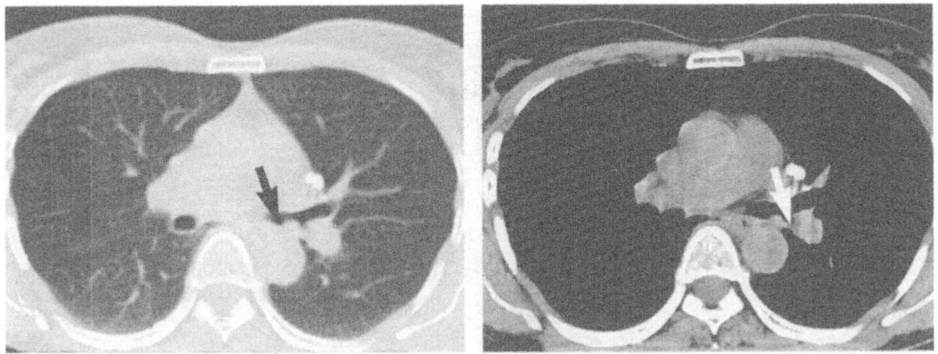

Fig. 34a, b. Endobronchial metastasis located on the posterior wall of the left main stem bronchus (*arrows*), originating from a *clear cell carcinoma of the kidney*

Approximately 26% of patients with diffuse pulmonary metastatic disease present with a picture of neoplastic micro- or macro-embolization of pulmonary vascularity (Fig. 35) [7]. Computed tomography may demonstrate multifocal beaded dilatation of the peripheral arteries, and multiple small peripheral infarct-like changes at the level of the secondary lobule with a mosaic pattern, especially when secondary to a microembolization from vascular or cardiac primary tumors [55].

Another peculiar pattern is the ground-glass consolidation with an air bronchogram inside. This may be secondary to a permeative diffusion through the air spaces, seen mostly in metastases from tumors of the gastrointestinal tract, in up to 10% of them [22].

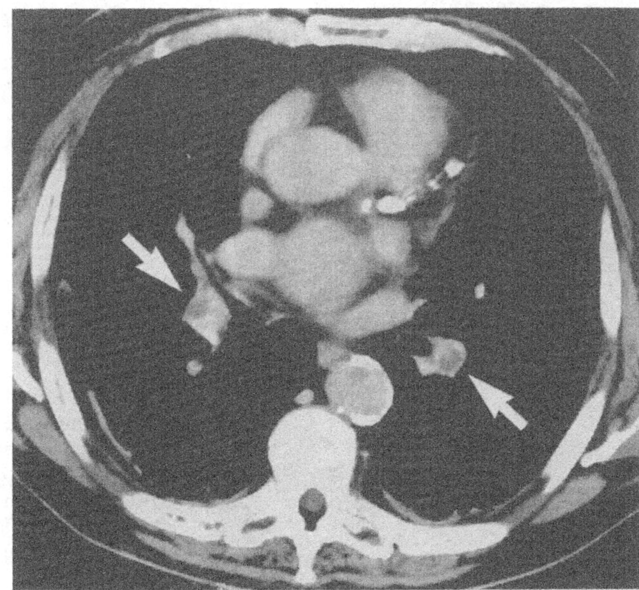

Fig. 35. Multiple neoplastic emboli (*arrows*) are identified within the lumen of the inferior lobar arteries bilaterally, secondary to a *clear cell carcinoma of the kidney*. The neoplastic nature of the thrombi was revealed at autopsy

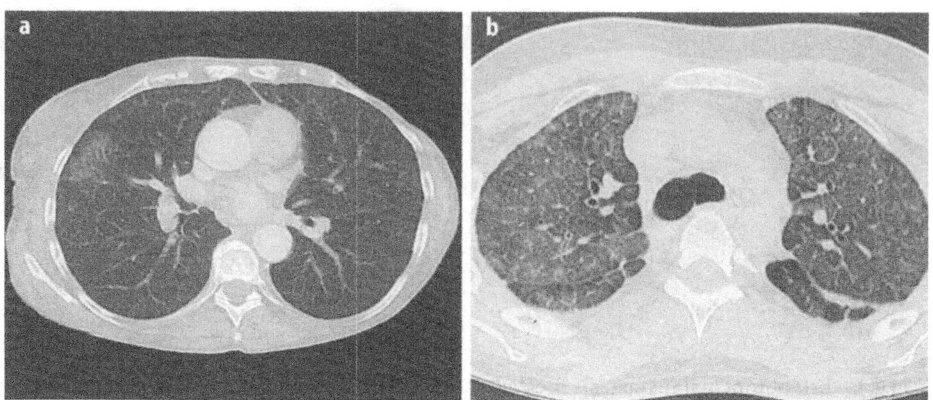

Fig. 36. a Focal lymphangitic carcinomatosis secondary to a *breast carcinoma.* **b** Diffuse atypical ground-glass carcinomatosis from a *gastric adenocarcinoma*

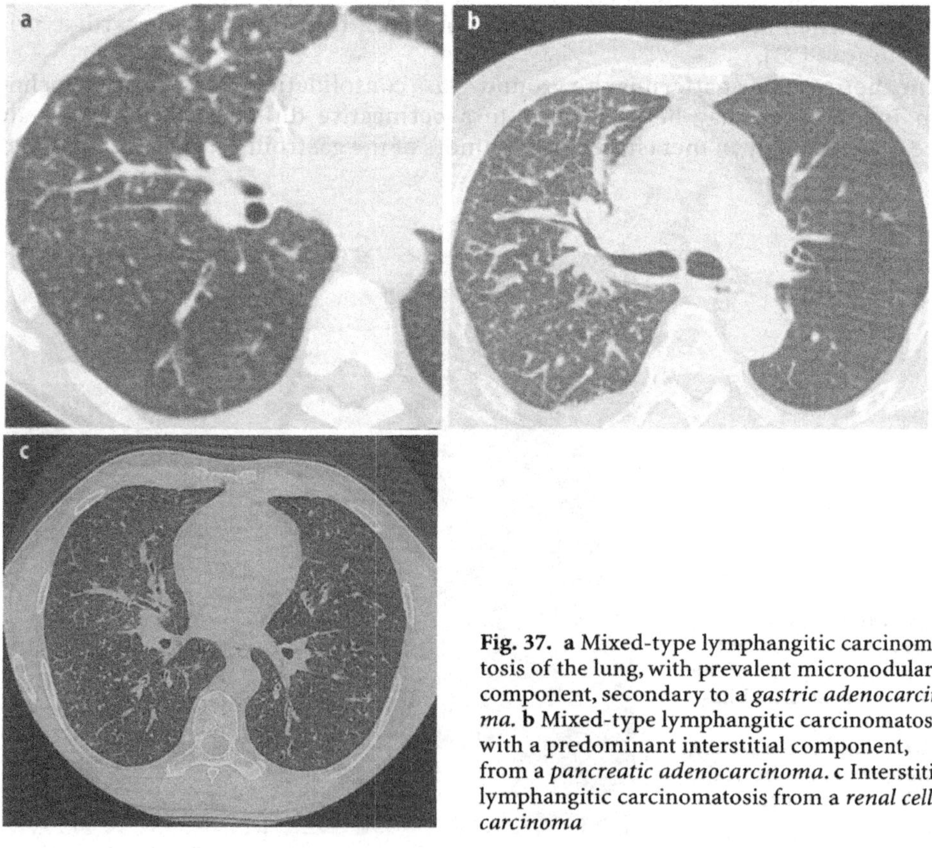

Fig. 37. a Mixed-type lymphangitic carcinomatosis of the lung, with prevalent micronodular component, secondary to a *gastric adenocarcinoma.* **b** Mixed-type lymphangitic carcinomatosis, with a predominant interstitial component, from a *pancreatic adenocarcinoma.* **c** Interstitial lymphangitic carcinomatosis from a *renal cell carcinoma*

Lymphangitic carcinomatosis is the consequence of a neoplastic growth which takes place within the lumen of the lymphatic vessels, secondary to a hematogenous spread through arterioles and capillaries, breech of the vascular walls, and invasion of the perivascular lymphatics [13, 55]. It is a relatively common phenomenon, seen in 6–8% of cases, although selected series have reported an incidence ranging from 24 to 56% [11, 12]. Approximately 80% of cases are due to adenocarcinomas, with the breast, stomach, and pancreas being the most common organs of origin [20]. Unlike nodular lesion which are exquisitely asymptomatic, lymphangitic carcinomatosis is often responsible for dyspnea and respiratory failure [55]. Computed tomography, especially with a high-resolution technique, is considered a prime diagnostic tool [11]; the latter is often the only technique which allows demonstration of the typical anatomic substrate of the carcinomatosis. The nodular or beaded thickening of the interstitial septa, otherwise absent in edema and fibrosis, the punctate central densities surrounded by polygonal thickening in 58% of cases and secondary to neoplastic proliferation within the interlobular septa and intralobular interstitium, and the absence of distortion or destruction of the normal lobular architecture, seen in fact in pulmonary fibrosis from which it can therefore be differentiated, are all diagnostic characteristics of this devastating entity [20]. The topographic prevalence of one of the interstitial components (subpleural, interlobular septal, peribronchovascular) is at the root of the variable CT appearance of the disease (Figs. 36, 37) [12]. Pulmonary edema, with its ill-defined contours and sarcoidosis, both characterized by less marked septal thickening and less frequent pleural effusions, may occasionally pose serious differential diagnostic problems [11, 20].

Finally, there are the so-called sterile metastases. During chemotherapy, especially in some highly chemosensitive histologic types, complete biologic resolution of a metastatic deposit is possible even in the presence of an anatomic residue [38]. Necrosis with or without fibrosis may justify the persistence of a pulmonary nodule or its decrease in size [39, 55] in the face of pathologically absent disease. There are no differentiating CT parameters [38]. Only demonstration of lack of evolution at follow-ups, in conjunction with a stable negativity of specific biologic markers when available (testicular germ cell tumors, gestational chorioncarcinomas) or a negative pathologic examination, may suggest the sterile nature of the nodule, when no other sites of disease are documented [55].

Pleura

The pleura is a frequent site of metastatic spread and hematogenous diffusion is the main route of colonization [7, 13, 28]. Adenocarcinomas, especially from the lung, breast, pancreas, and stomach, are the most frequently responsible primary tumors [20, 38]. Furthermore, the pleura is the most important and earliest site of metastatic diffusion from invasive thymomas [20].

At CT the typical appearance is of plaque lesions of variable dimensions, generally multifocal and with contrast enhancement, extending to both pulmonary and mediastinal pleural leaflets [12, 38]. A diffuse involvement of the whole hemithorax is occasionally detected, similar to a mesothelioma, as seen, for example, in pleural localizations from a renal cell carcinoma (Fig. 38) [55]. These lesions, in relation to

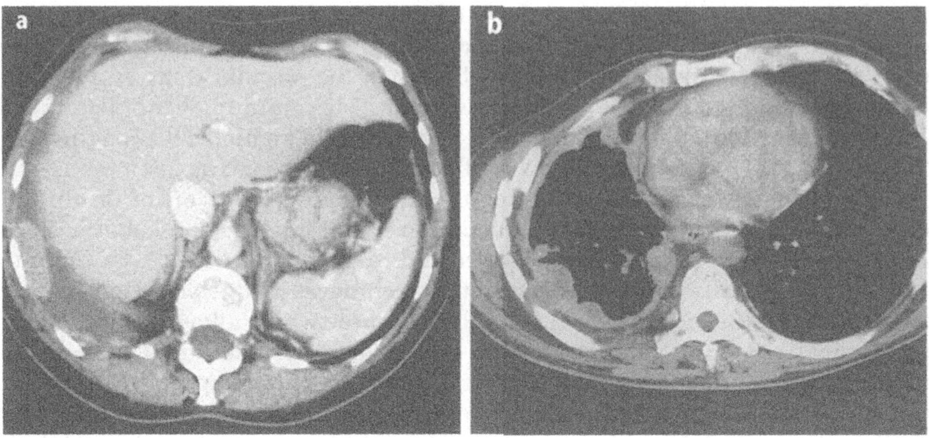

Fig. 38. Metastatic pleural tumors from *breast carcinomas,* with **a** en plaque morphology or **b** diffusely infiltrating

the inherent hypervascularity of the primary tumors, exhibit marked contrast enhancement (Fig. 39). A pleural effusion is frequently associated with metastatic deposits of the pleura, especially in carcinomas of the breast and of the ovary [20]. In particular, it is not unusual to detect a malignant pleural effusion without focal nodularities at CT along the course of ovarian carcinomas. Lymphatic extension through the diaphragmatic peritoneum, the plexus of the pleural surface of the diaphragm itself, and the lymphatic connections through the mediastinum account for the relatively high incidence of such lesions [1, 7].

The differential diagnosis entails a long series of predominantly inflammatory/ infectious processes, particularly tuberculosis and fungal colonizations, infarcts, and congestive heart failure [37, 55].

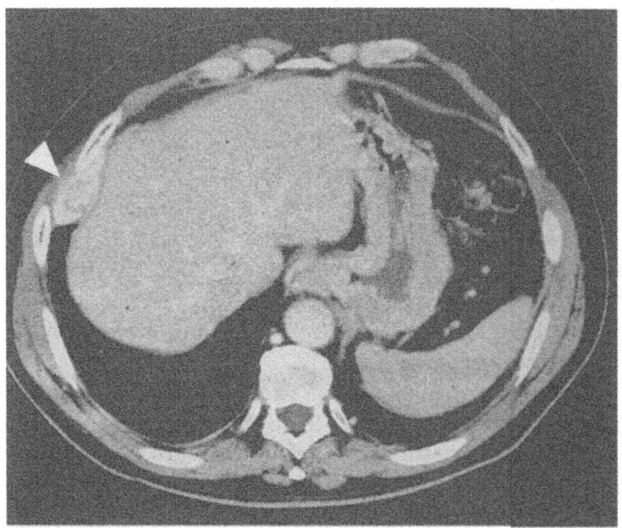

Fig. 39. Hypervascular pleural metastasis, from a *renal cell carcinoma,* characterized by marked contrast enhancement (*arrowhead*)

Liver

The liver is the second site of metastatic diffusion in order of frequency [20, 53] Gastrointestinal, pancreatic, cholecystic, mammary, and pulmonary neoplasms represent the primary tumors which most often diffuse to this organ [1]. Sarcomas, melanomas, as well as renal and thyroidal carcinomas are somewhat less frequently observed [7, 20].

The peculiar vascular anatomy of the liver, sustained by the hepatic artery for 20–25% and for 75–80% by the portal venous system, significantly affects the detectability of hepatic lesions during contrast enhanced CT [63]. Since the vast majority of metastases recruit systemic arterial vascularization for their blood supply, it is indispensable to tailor the contrast bolus injection and the CT data acquisition to obtain optimal arterial-phase imaging, in order to maximize the density gradient between the lesions themselves and the surrounding parenchyma. It is in fact possible to see rapid homogenization of the parenchymal density, during the following portal venous phase, which may therefore mask underlying small lesions. The newest CT scanners, with helical technology, allow imaging of the entire organ in both vascular phases; thus, the sensitivity has improved markedly [65]. The spatial resolution, however, is still suboptimal for adequate evaluation of lesions measuring less than 10 mm. Some authors have in fact advocated the use of helical CT after selective catheterization of the hepatic artery, or of the celiac/superior mesenteric artery, in order to maximize the difference in contrast during the arterial phase [66].

The CT appearance of hepatic metastases is variable and depends primarily on the dimensions, vascularization, structure, and degree of necrosis of the lesion itself, as well as on the amount and mode of administration of the intravenous iodinated contrast [63]. In the presence of multiple metastases (as in mammary or colic carcinomas), lesions may exhibit variable appearance and enhancement within the same patient. On the other hand, metastases from differing primary tumors may exhibit similar features at CT [67].

At *baseline non-enhanced CT* studies, metastatic lesions appear most often hypodense with sometimes confluent nodules and typically ill-defined contours (Fig. 40)

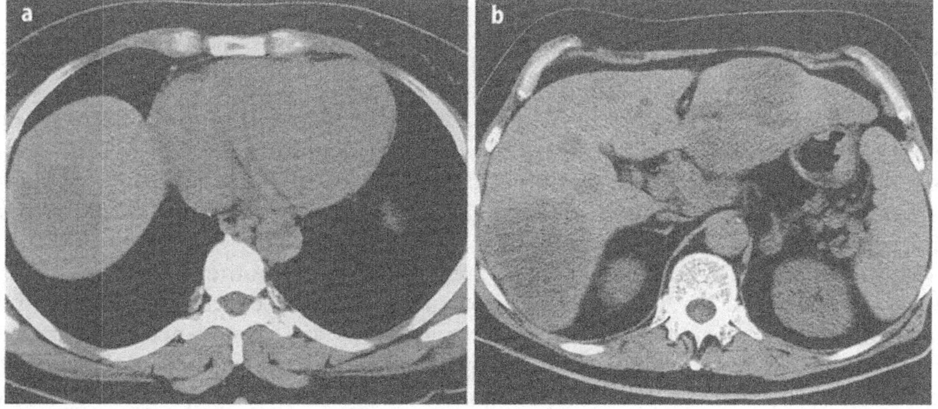

Fig. 40. Hypodense hepatic metastases from *bronchogenic carcinomas*, with **a** a nodular or **b** confluent appearance

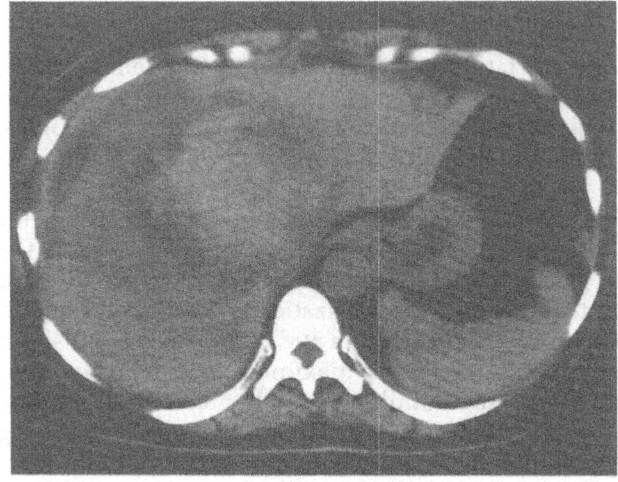

Fig. 41. Subacute hemorrhage in a metastatic *melanoma*

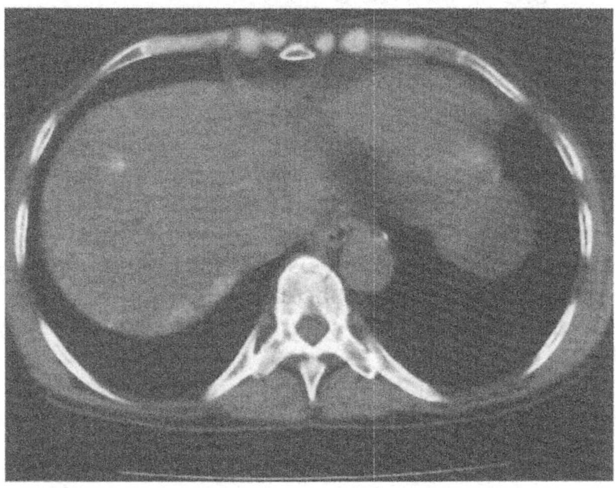

Fig. 42. "Dusty" calcifications within a diffuse metastatic process, secondary to a *mucoid adenocarcinoma of the stomach*

[63, 67]. Only when in the presence of an acute/subacute hemorrhagic component (generally in hypervascular tumors), or when occurring within a diffusely and markedly steatotic hepatic parenchyma, will metastases appear relatively or absolutely hyperdense in comparison with the background (Fig. 41) [42, 67–69]. Also, the presence of diffuse "dusty" calcifications or of large lesions with high cellularity may cause the density to be slightly superior to the surrounding normal hepatic parenchyma (Fig. 42) [67, 26].

Not infrequently, hypodense necrotic areas, with values sometimes close to the values of water (HU 0–20), are seen, involving either site central portion or the totality of the metastatic lesion [24]. Much rarer is a cystic appearance of the metastatic focus, generally secondary to cystic primary malignancies such as those from the ovary or the pancreas. Also rare is a lipoid component, with negative HU values and seen typically in metastases from primary tumors normally exhibiting this feature, such as immature teratomas and liposarcomas [23, 29].

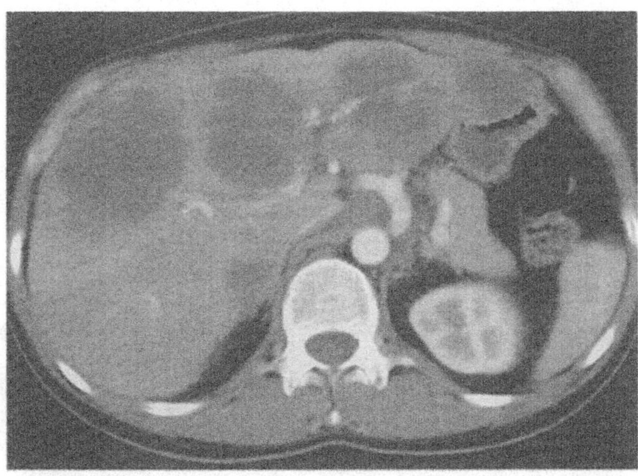

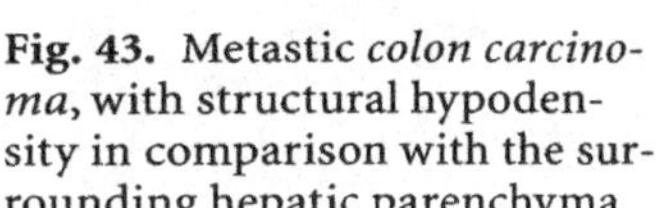

Fig. 43. Metastic *colon carcinoma*, with structural hypodensity in comparison with the surrounding hepatic parenchyma

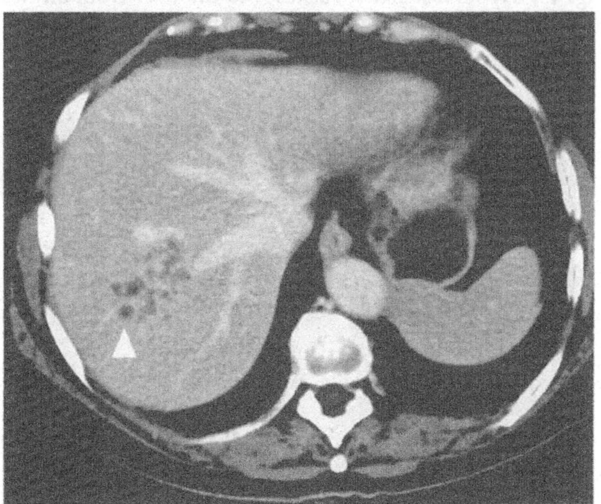

Fig. 44. Cluster of multiple hepatic metastases from a *bronchogenic carcinoma*. Some of the lesions demonstrate a thin peripheral rim of marked contrast enhancement

After intravenous contrast medium administration, lesion enhancement, variable in relation to the type of lesion and its degree of vascularization, may exhibit five different patterns: *scarce or not otherwise detectable*, with structures that remain persistently hypodense in relation to the surrounding parenchyma (Fig. 43); *marked, ring-like*, with peripheral enhancement particularly well demonstrated in the early arterial phases (Fig. 44); *marked, global enhancement*, with a rapid washout, hyperdensity in the arterial phase, and isodensity in the portal venous phase, typical of tumors with a high degree of vascularization (Fig. 45); *progressive centripetal enhancement*, hemangioma-like, with occasional delayed hyperdensity, more typically seen in breast cancers (Fig. 46); *delayed mild to moderate* enhancement, often detected only after several hours from the initial injection of contrast, seen more often in pseudocystic lesions (Fig. 47) [23, 63, 64, 67, 69–71].

The differential diagnosis of hepatic metastases is extremely complex in relation to the number, morphology, dimension, and enhancement of the lesions. It includes cystic lesions, hemangiomas, lymphomas, hepatocellular carcinomas, and chol-

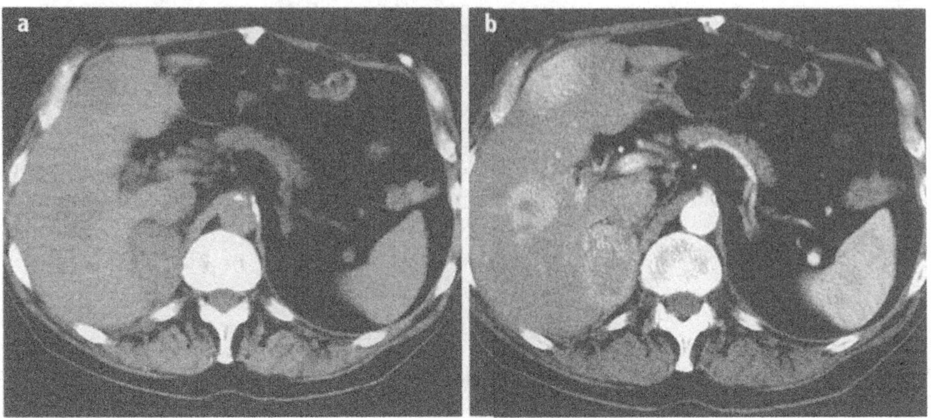

Fig. 45. Hypervascular metastases to the liver from an *ileal carcinoid,* **a** at baseline and **b** after intravenous contrast administration. There is concurrent involvement of the right adrenal gland

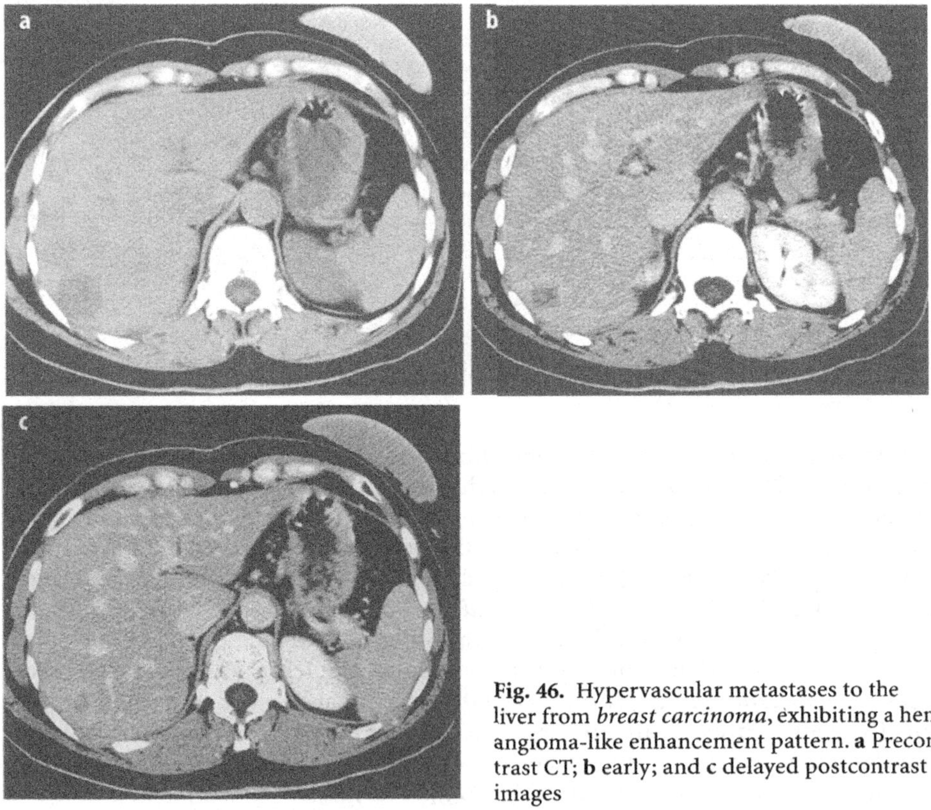

Fig. 46. Hypervascular metastases to the liver from *breast carcinoma,* exhibiting a hemangioma-like enhancement pattern. **a** Precontrast CT; **b** early; and **c** delayed postcontrast images

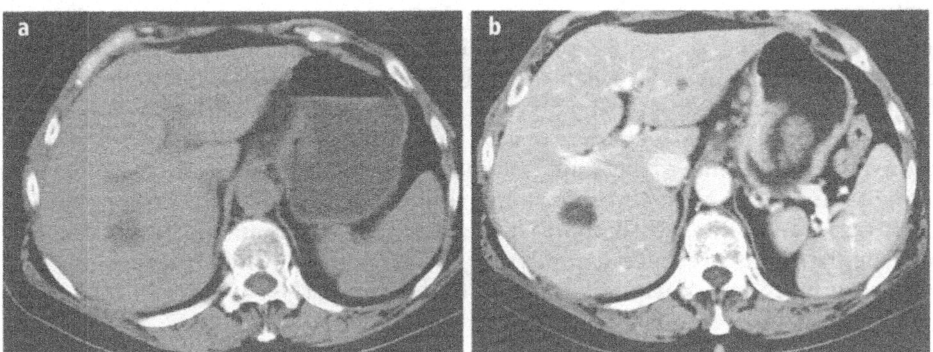

Fig. 47. Hepatic metastasis from a *gastric carcinoma*, cystic in appearance, **a** at baseline and **b** post-contrast scanning

angiocarcinomas [63, 67]. Careful assessment of densitometric parameters and structural features metastases, thin collimation to minimize volume averaging artifacts, implementation of clinical and historical data, and evaluation of synchronous signs are all aspects which may aid in the differential diagnosis.

One particular pattern of metastatic disease of the liver which deserves specific mention is lymphangitic diffusion. This takes the form of dilatation of the lymphatic ducts in the perivascular spaces, with infiltration of the portal spaces and secondary fibrosis. The CT appearance is characterized by ill-defined and irregularly contoured hypodense lesions, with a tendency to follow a vascular distribution, which may sometimes be associated with segmental dilatation of the intra-hepatic biliary ducts [16].

Adrenal Glands

The adrenal glands are one of the most frequent sites of metastases, probably the most frequent site if one considers their weight in relation to other organs [20]. The high concentration of molecules inhibiting the immunologic response present in the adrenal cortex, such as the steroid hormone present in this location, along with the presence of a large number of arterio-venous anastomoses in this organ, probably account for these glands being so prone to metastatic involvement [72]. Depending on histologic subtype, adrenal lesions are observed in 10–20% of cases at the time of staging and in 35–40% at autopsy [20]. Bronchogenic carcinoma is the primary malignancy which most frequently metastastizes to the adrenal glands. Other responsible primary tumors are breast, renal, cutaneous (melanoma), gastro-intestinal, pancreatic, and hepatic neoplasms [44, 69, 72].

Adrenal lesions, which are bilateral in approximately 60% of cases, are clinically silent, even when voluminous, because only minimal amounts of surviving endocrine tissue are necessary to maintain the metabolic and saline homeostasis. It is believed that hypofunctioning syndromes may be more frequent, but that they are masked by the effects of antitumoral chemotherapy, often including corticosteroid medications, or go otherwise unrecognized because of the non-specific nature of their symptoms in neoplastic patients [72].

The CT appearance is again highly variable and may comprise aspects characterized by an enlarged gland with preservation of its normal morphology and homogeneous density, especially when the lesions are small. As metastatic lesions grow the gland may lose its shape and be substituted by an oval mass, with progressively heterogeneous density due to necrosis or hemorrhage. Occasionally, with very large lesions, the entire gland may appear hypodense, which is seen often in metastatic colon cancer because of necrosis or mucin secretion (Fig. 48) [72]. After intravenous administration of iodinated contrast medium, enhancement is always present to some degree. This presence is moderate and irregular in the larger lesions and it may be limited to the peripheral portion of the tumor (Fig. 49) [72].

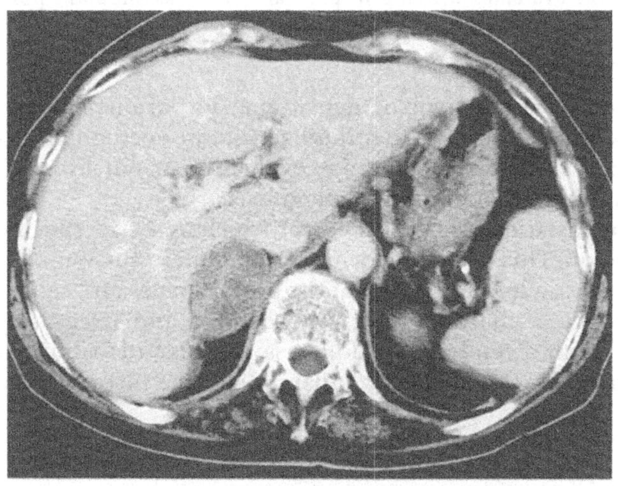

Fig. 48. Right adrenal metastatic tumor originating from a *bronchogenic carcinoma*, oval in shape, demonstrating markedly heterogeneous structure due to necrotic and hemorrhagic phenomena

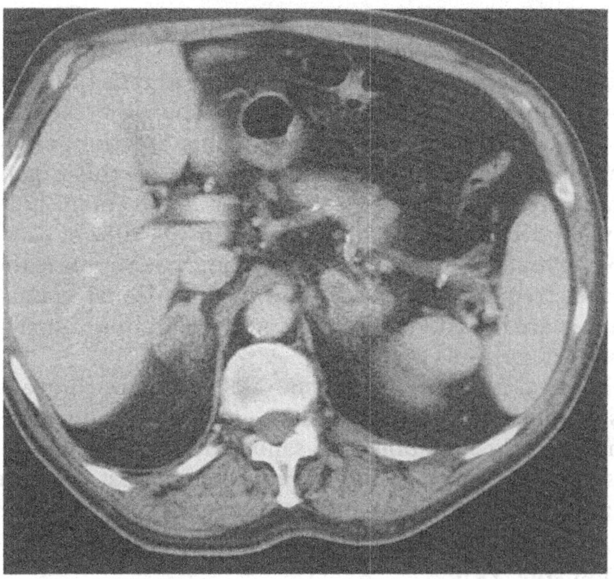

Fig. 49. Bilateral adrenal metastases from *bronchogenic carcinoma*, with a typical peripheral rim of enhancement, after intravenous contrast administration

Irregular contours with soft tissue strands radiating from the surface of the gland are the expression of a transcapsular diffusion of the neoplastic disease. Intratumoral calcifications are infrequent and are generally associated to mucin-producing gastro-intestinal tumors or to psammomatous papillary carcinomas, as well as to post-chemotherapy [23]. Hemorrhagic complications are also rare [41], generally secondary to renal cell carcinomas or other hypervascular tumors [45]. Hemorrhages may evolve into large retroperitoneal hematomas, with densities obviously varying according to the age of the hemorrhagic event, just as seen in the intraglandular collections [43].

Unilateral metastases must be differentiated primarily from a non-hyperfunctioning adenoma. A metastasis more frequently exhibits higher density at baseline (≥ 30 HU), contrast enhancement, heterogeneous structure, irregular contours, and dimensions larger than 3 cm [72].

The presence of strictly adipose foci within an adrenal nodule, although always viewed as virtually pathognomonic of myelolipoma, may in fact be secondary to a metastatic lesion which, in its extracapsular expansion toward the surrounding soft tissues, may engulf the periglandular fat, thus producing discrete misleading hypodense foci [73].

Lesions of other nature, such as pseudocysts, hematomas, inflammatory lesions or collections, as well as benign and malignant primary neoplasms, may, from time to time, represent the potential source of diagnostic dilemmas. In *bilateral disease*, adrenal hyperplasia, granulomatous inflammatory diseases, hemorrhage, and the much rarer lymphomatous localizations are the principal diagnostic alternatives. Whereas hyperplasia will again appear as mostly hypodense, with no significant enhancement or glandular distortion, tuberculosis, coccidioidomycosis, histoplasmosis, and toxoplasmosis may be differentiated in their florid phase due to clinical and laboratory data. Hemorrhages can be suspected due to knowledge of specific underlying diatheses, anticoagulation therapy, and recent traumatic or surgical events [72]. Finally, lymphomatous localizations tend to be homogeneous in density, with much rarer necrosis and scant contrast enhancement, and are often accompanied by other synchronous nodal or organ lesions [74, 75].

Peritoneum

The peritoneum is a frequent site of metastatic involvement [20]. The mesothelial superficial lining appears to be very vulnerable to colonization by neoplastic cells, which adhere to it and proliferate, thus forming flat foci of infiltration or nodules. These may in turn shed other neoplastic cells into the serous cavity [1, 7]. Permeation of the subserosal lymphatics also plays a relevant role in the colonization process. The irritating stimulus generated by the tumoral implants generates ascites, which in turn favors the diffusion of tumoral cells and their subsequent implant on other serosal surfaces, such as the pouch of Douglas, ovaries, omentum, and the diaphragmatic peritoneum. There is a specific direction of circulation of peritoneal fluid, governed by gravitational factors, variations of the intra-abdominal pressure, and by intestinal peristalsis; therefore, the preferential locations for metastatic implants coincide with those where the ascitic flow slows or arrests [1].

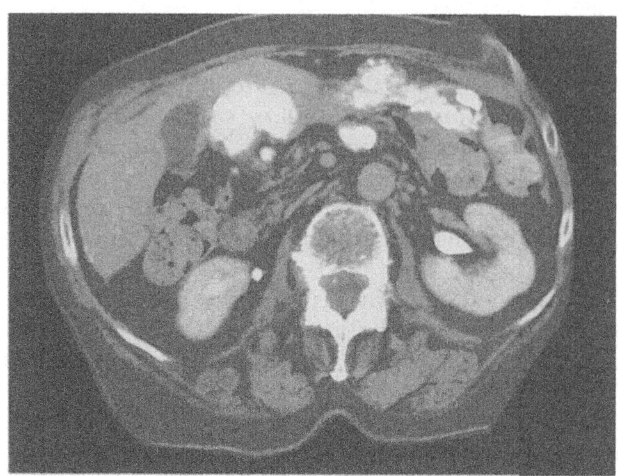

Fig. 50. Calcified omental metastases from a *serous papillary cystadenocarcinoma of the ovary*

In any neoplasm at an advanced stage, infiltration of the serosal membranes may take place with further diffusion of the tumor itself [7]. Tumors that typically cause a miliary diffusion in the peritoneum are ovarian (occasionally with calcific foci; Fig. 50), gastro-intestinal, pancreatic, and breast neoplasms [1]. The CT appearance is characterized by a massive infiltration with *omental caking* or *multiple nodules* of extremely variable size, both enhancing after contrast medium administration. These appearances are associated with thickened peritoneal leaflets and irregular hyperdense curved strands which focally or diffusely obliterate the peritoneal adipose tissue (Fig. 51). Not infrequently, involvement of the serosal surface appears as marginal irregularities of the walls of viscera which may also be thickened [29], or with contrast-enhancing areas (Fig. 52). It is helpful to remember that, especially during follow-up of patients undergoing chemotherapy for ovarian carcinoma, the peritoneum statistically represents, along with the liver, the most frequent site of recurrence of disease [7, 76]. When evaluating for tiny peritoneal lesions, thin (4–5 mm) section CT with bolus injection of contrast is mandatory [77].

Microfoci of steatonecrosis and/or fibrotic changes of the peritoneum, often secondary to prior chemotherapy (especially with intraperitoneal infusion), represent the most important differential diagnosis. Some clues may be gathered only by the chronology of lesions and comparative evaluation of specific serum markers such as the CA-125 [76, 77]. Furthermore, in patients with a history of multiple chemotherapy cycles, recurrence of disease may not be associated with the otherwise usual ascites.

A particular and rare occurrence, often the source of diagnostic difficulties, may be represented by the so-called pseudomyxoma peritonei. This is the result of a massive peritoneal colonization (through rupture or direct metastatic implants) by a low-grade mucinous epithelial neoplasm, originating from the ovary, appendix, pancreas, and gallbladder. Cases secondary to tumors of the uterus, urachus, or omphalo-mesenteric duct have also been described [7, 17]. The CT appearance takes the form of a massive peritoneal infiltration by a hypodense mass, with HU values of 10–35. Sometimes these may appear more solid with fluid–fluid levels and

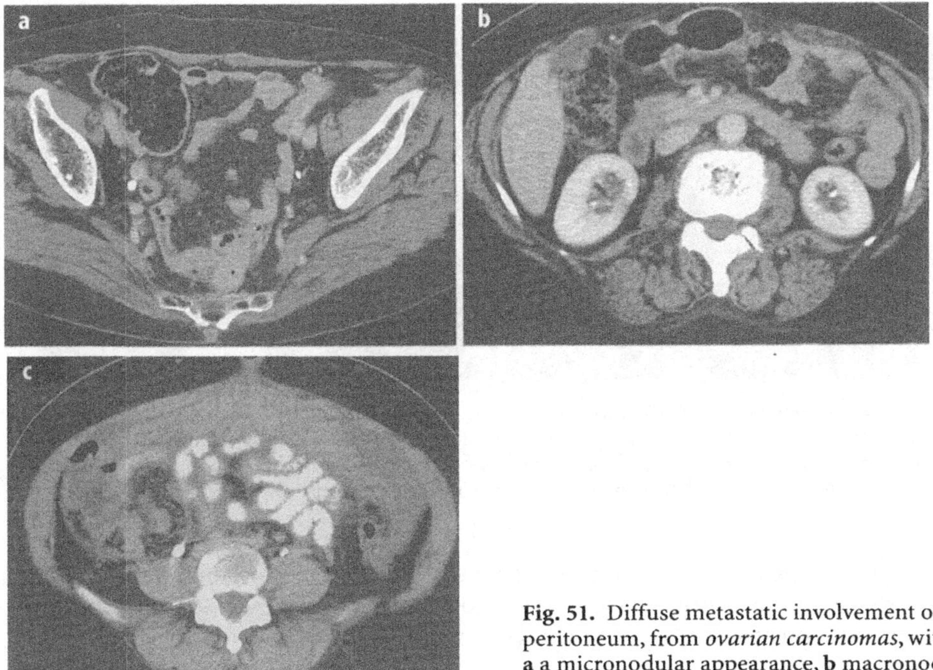

Fig. 51. Diffuse metastatic involvement of the peritoneum, from *ovarian carcinomas*, with **a** a micronodular appearance, **b** macronodular lesions, and with **c** "omental cake"

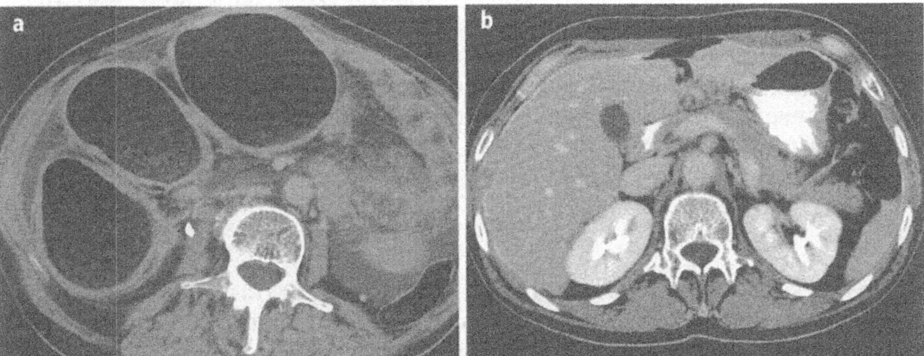

Fig. 52. **a** Peritoneal metastases from *ovarian carcinoma*, demonstrating extensive involvement of the serosal surface of multiple ileal loops, with secondary chronic partial intestinal obstruction and irregular thickening of the visceral walls. **b** Diffuse carcinomatosis of the hepatic capsule, appearing as a diffuse and regular contrast enhancement of the liver surface, secondary to an *endometrioid carcinoma of the ovary*

septa, or as large hypodense nodules with thickened and enhancing contours (Fig. 53) [18]. Calcifications of the nodules are not rare. The masses typically cause extrinsic indentation of the hepatic, or seldom splenic, surfaces, with a concave appearance of the capsules [78]. The intestinal loops are typically displaced in the lateral abdominal quadrants by these gelatinous masses, unlike what is seen with ascites where the displacement occurs medially [29]. In the early stages the dif-

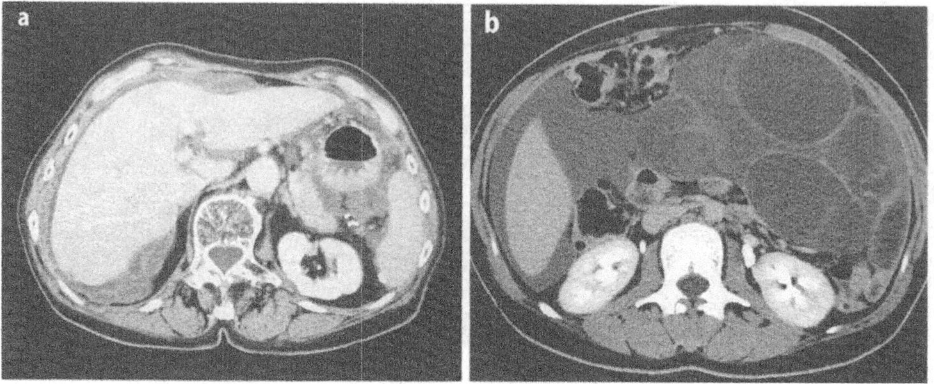

Fig. 53. Pseudomyxoma peritoneii. **a** *Mucinous cystadenocarcinoma of the ovary* causing massive peritoneal infiltration, with fluid and/or markedly low density, as well as multiple intralesional septa. **b** *mucinous adenocarcinoma of the gallbladder* generating multiple large masses in the peritoneum, characterized by markedly thickened walls, intralesional septa, and small vegetations

ferential diagnosis includes peritonitis from tuberculosis or pyogenic bacteria. The large nodules are discriminated from pseudocysts and other extra-pancreatic fluid collections if a positive history of prior pancreatitis is elicited, or from disseminated hydatid disease [78].

It is worth mentioning that the abdominal ligaments and the peritoneal folds, representing the anatomic infrastructure for intraperitoneal organs and their vascular, lymphatic, and nervous pathways, may also constitute a bi-directional route of connection between the abdomen and the pelvis, and between the intra- and retroperitoneal spaces, offering preformed paths of tumoral diffusion. This may explain the transperitoneal extension of tumors which otherwise do not normally involve the peritoneum [79, 80].

Bone

Despite that fact the bone receives only a small (5 – 10 %) fraction of the cardiac output, it represents one of the most typical targets of metastatic involvement. Approximately 32 % of patients with a malignant neoplasm develop skeletal metastases in the course of their disease [81]. Their incidence, however, rises to approximately 70 % in patients with breast or prostate carcinomas which, along with renal, bronchogenic, bladder, and thyroidal neoplasms, represent the histologic types most frequently responsible for these lesions [20]. In the pediatric population neuroblastomas, osseous sarcomas, and leukemia are the tumors most frequently metastasizing to the skeleton [81, 82].

Diffusion of disease to the skeleton is virtually always hematogenous [83], through the arterial tree, and the red marrow represents the target element of such metastatization [1]. The skeletal segments, statistically most frequent sites of involvement are in fact those in which red marrow is more widely represented. Within the red marrow, the walls of the capillary sinusoids demonstrate fenestrations and discontinuities [7]. This probably represents the main reason for which metastatization in segments of bones affected by post-radiation changes is practically exceptional [82].

The vertebrae, by virtue of the particular anastomoses present between the perivertebral and the intraosseous venous plexus, are a typical anatomic location for bony metastases [84]. In 5–10% of cases signs of associated marrow invasion or compression of the nervous roots are identified [84]. Ribs, sternum, pelvis, as well as skull and long bones, particularly the proximal humeri and femurs, are other frequent locations, in decreasing order of frequency [82].

The majority of lesions develop in the cancellous bone, although in later phases involvement of the cortex and of the subperiosteal region is possible [7].

In prostatic and mammary carcinomas diffusion through the venous route is particularly significant. Increase in intra-abdominal pressure may cause temporary inversion of the direction of blood flow from the caval venous system toward the vertebral veins with subsequent early involvement of the thoracolumbar spine and of the pelvis [7, 10].

Numerous other factors have been advocated to play a role in the pathogenesis of the metastatic process, such as prostaglandins, osteoblast-, and osteoclast-activating factors. These may govern the evolution of lesions toward lytic or blastic character [5]. Osteoblastic metastases are generally associated with prostate tumors (80–90%), mammary carcinomas (especially after treatment), lymphomas [82, 85], carcinoids, mucinous tumors of the gastrointestinal tract, osteosarcomas, and retinoblastomas. The shift to sclerotic character of an otherwise lytic metastasis may be the result of a positive response to antitumoral therapy. Initially, a sclerotic rim may be detected which then progresses toward the center of the lesion, occasionally causing a true eburnation [37, 85]. Conversely, lytic changes appearing within a sclerotic metastasis may indicate progression of disease [85]. A well-known and frequent complication of skeletal metastases is represented by the occurrence of pathologic fractures [81, 84].

Computed tomography generally demonstrates areas of osseous destruction with infiltrating and ill-defined contours, heterogeneously hypodense structure, and mild contrast enhancement (Fig. 54). Extension to and through the cortex may

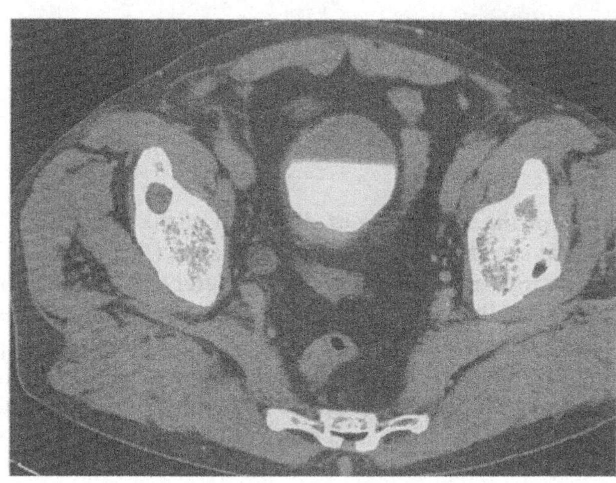

Fig. 54. Osteolytic metastasis from *bladder carcinoma*, localized in the right acetabulum and characterized by destruction and substitution of the cancellous bone by a soft tissue nodule, without involvement of the bony cortex

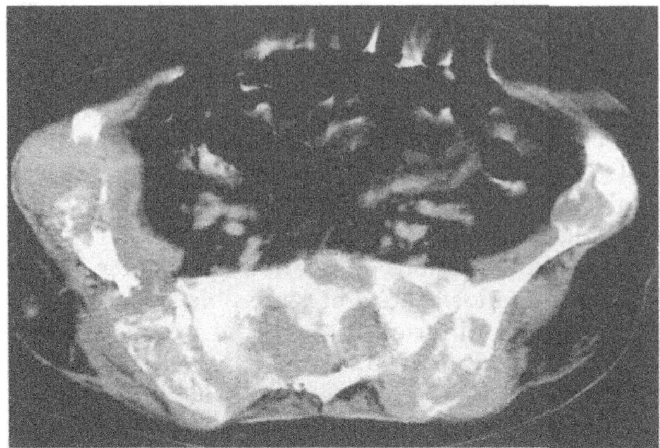

Fig. 55. Osteolytic metastasis from *breast carcinoma*, causing diffuse bony destruction and massive infiltration of the cortex leading to diffusion to the extraskeletal soft tissues

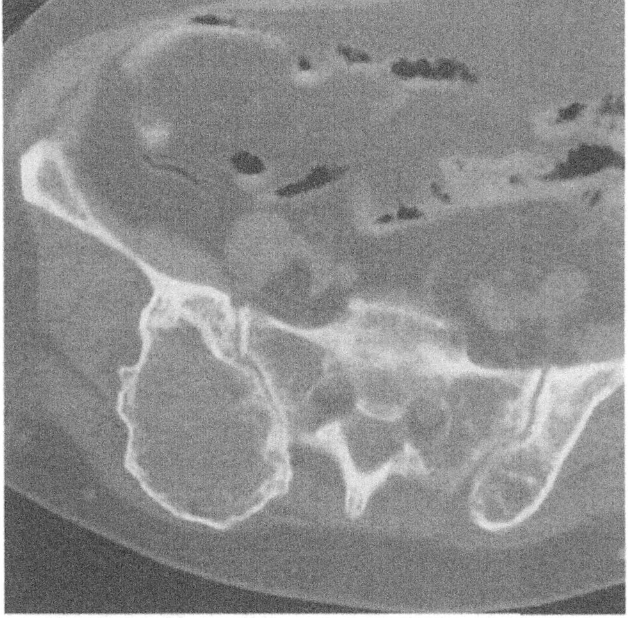

Fig. 56. Solitary osteolytic metastasis of the right ilium from *hepatic cell carcinoma*, with ballooning of the cortex due to marked expansion of its intramedullary component and with a myeloma-like appearance

represent the first stage of diffusion of the secondary tumor to the soft tissues and adjacent striated muscles and fat planes (Fig. 55) [82]. Areas of calcification and/or ossification may occasionally be detected in the paraskeletal soft tissue masses which actually represent islands of bones displaced, destroyed, and infiltrated by the expanding tumoral masses [81]. Selected histologic types, such as those originating from the liver, kidney, or thyroid, are associated with a marked expansion of the medullary component, with a myeloma-like appearance (Fig. 56). Other tumors, namely prostate, lung, and gastrointestinal cancers, as well as neuroblastomas, elicit a prominent periosteal reaction. Tumors with a slower replication rate are generally

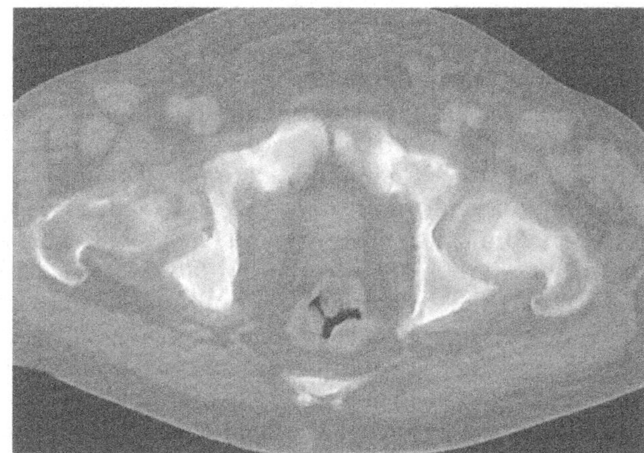

Fig. 57. Osteoblastic metastic diffusion to the axial skeleton, from *prostate carcinoma*

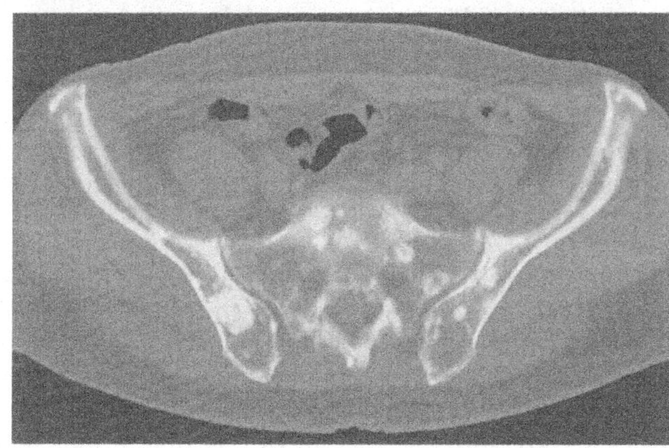

Fig. 58. Multiple osteoblastic metastases from *prostate carcinoma*, characterized by multiple foci of sclerosis within the substance of the cancellous bone

characterized by better definition of their contours, delimited by a reactive peripheral sclerotic rim [86].

Among osteoblastic forms, CT may reveal a diffuse global involvement of the anatomic segment in question (Fig. 57). On other occasions the lesion may appear exquisitely focal, involving only the cancellous portion of the bone (Fig. 58).

Lymph Nodes

Neoplastic diffusion to lymph nodes represents one of the most significant prognostic parameters, influencing the survival of the neoplastic patients and their therapeutic management [87]. The negative impact upon the surgical resectability of non-small cell lung cancers in the presence of disease extending to mediastinal nodal stations is a well-known fact, accounting for a drastic reduction in the life expectancy in this scenario [8, 88]. Similarly, assessment of extension of disease to the axillary lymph nodes of breast carcinomas represents the main predictor of the risk of relapse in patients treated with otherwise radical intent [8].

Knowledge of the specific routes of lymphatic drainage is of paramount importance in evaluating the extent of disease, especially in relation to the distance between the primary site and the nodal filters of first order [5]. It is also important to remember that any form of obstruction of the lymphatic drainage may cause metastases to skip one or more expected nodal stations, or even cause retrograde diffusion due to inversion of the lymphatic flow [7].

At imaging, short-axis *dimension*, normally ranging from 8 to 12 mm depending on the anatomic district, represents the most important parameter of suspicion for a metastatic lymphadenopathy [87–90]. More recently, a new parameter has been advocated in the evaluation of lymph node involvement, represented by the ratio between the longitudinal and axial diameters of the node itself [87]. Consequently, values higher than 2 would have to be considered indicative of hyperplastic enlargement, whereas a ratio less than 2 is highly suspicious for metastatic disease. These conclusions are based on the idea that hyperplastic lymph nodes, although enlarged, tend to retain their original oval elongated morphology, whereas nodes containing neoplastic tissue, which notoriously exhibits radial growth, have a spherical appearance [87, 90].

On the other hand, *structural characteristics* of lymph nodes only rarely provide additional and more specific elements of diagnosis [91]. The exception is represented by lymphadenopathy of the head and neck region where the presence of central necrosis, in the form of foci of heterogeneous hypodensity, virtually always characterizes a metastatic lesion (Fig. 59) [87, 91]. The differential diagnosis embraces the adipose hilar metaplasia, generally resulting from chronic inflammatory processes and for the most part identified at the periphery of the node [90]. Detection of negative HU values, especially with the aid of thin (2–3 mm) sections, may offer an additional differential clue [87]. A strictly necrotic nodal structure is rarely detected in the absence of a prior chemotherapy treatment (Fig. 60).

At all levels considered, however, the well-known limitations of CT remain: the *false-positive* findings, related to enlarged nodes which are otherwise the site of

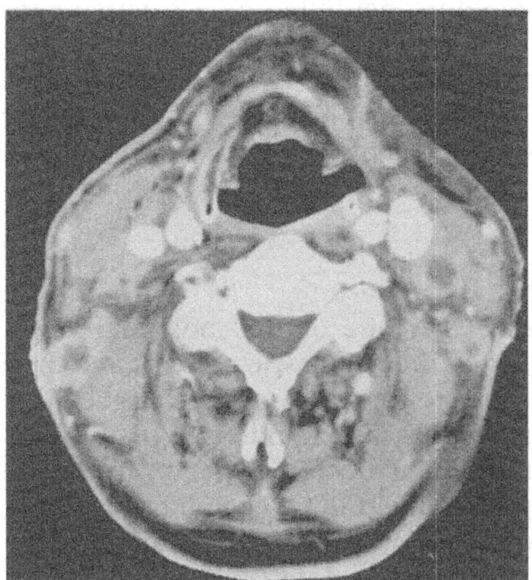

Fig. 59. Lymph node metastases from a *squamous cell carcinoma of the maxillary sinus,* which demonstrates areas of heterogenous hypodensity due to central necrosis

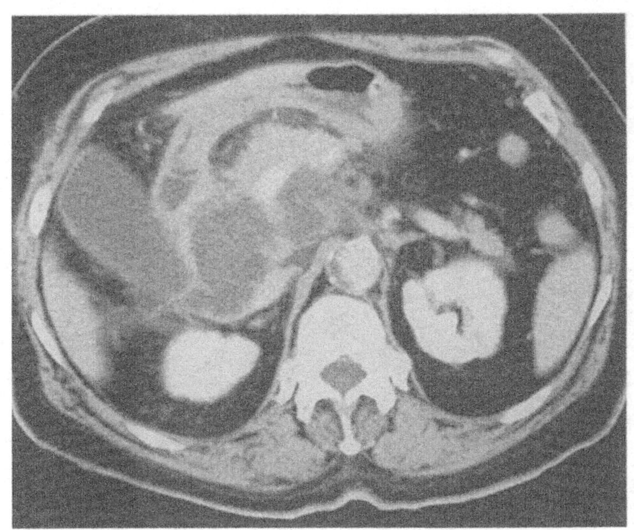

Fig. 60. Large metastatic deposits to the lymph nodes of the retroperitoneum with a diffusely hypodense structure due to extensive necrosis and secondary to a *colon carcinoma*

reactive changes or inflammatory/infectious processes (cat-scratch disease, tuberculosis, sarcoidosis, histoplasmosis) [88, 90], as well as the *false-negative* results, which occur in the presence of microscopic metastatic deposits which do not alter the volume, contour, or structure of the lymph node [89, 91].

The lack of specificity of the CT findings is at the root of the frequent necessity for lymphadenectomy and subsequent histopathologic analysis as a diagnostic tool in numerous tumors [10].

Detection of *extracapsular diffusion* of tumoral tissue is characteristic and of great prognostic value. This finding is detected in approximately 74% of lymph nodes displaying a diameter greater than 3 cm [90, 91]. Tumoral extension beyond

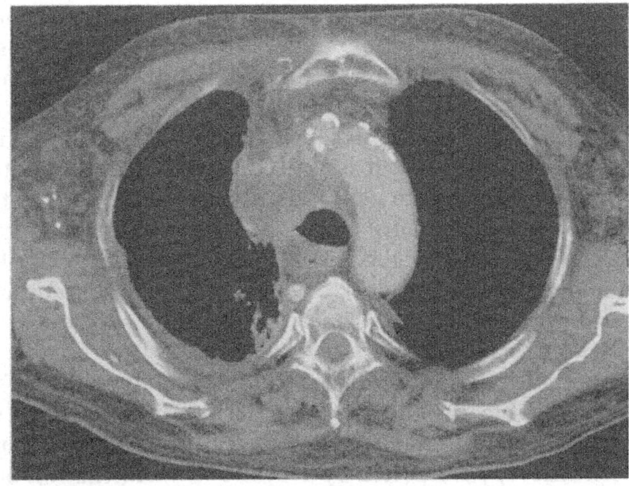

Fig. 61. Mediastinal carcinomatosis from *gastric carcinoma*

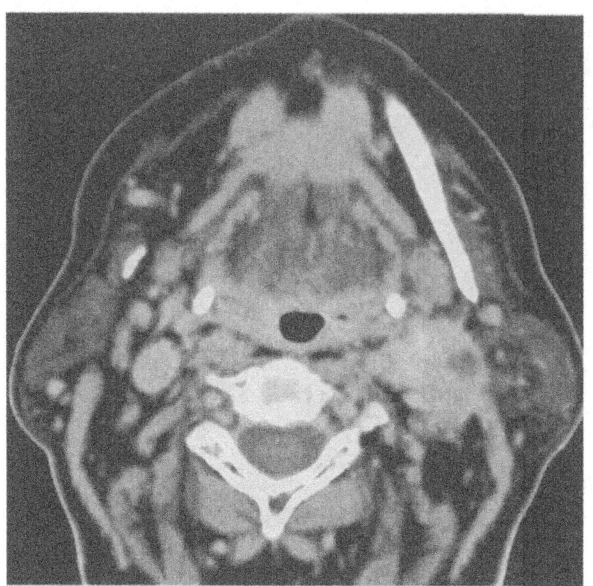

Fig. 62. Nodal metastasis, from *squamous cell carcinoma of the oral cavity*, with diffuse extra-capsular diffusion and involvement of the jugulo-carotid vascular bundle

the border of the nodal capsule causes obliteration of the surrounding adipose planes, which in turn appear marked by thick contrast-enhancing striations, curvilinear or serpiginous, which may even exhibit the appearance of a massive carcinosis, in which the adipose tissue is totally effaced by hypodense or solid tissue (Fig. 61) [87, 91]. The less than massive appearance may indeed also be seen during infectious processes, as well as in cases of recent irradiation or surgical manipulation [90].

It is also important to assess possible *infiltration of the loco-regional vascular trunks* (Fig. 62). Involvement of the arterio-venous pedicles, such as the jugulo-carotid or mesenteric axis, as a consequence of transcapsular extension of the tumor, deeply affects prognosis, especially in view of a possible surgical approach [9, 87, 90]. If the vessel appears surrounded for more than 50 % of its circumference by the pathologic lymph node, infiltration of the vascular wall may be reliably presumed. If the contact is otherwise limited to a small focus, direct invasion is unlikely.

Another parameter deserving careful assessment is *contrast enhancement* of the lymph node [90]. It is well known that nodal metastases from hypervascular primary tumors, such as Kaposi's sarcomas as well as thyroidal and renal carcinomas, may occasionally replicate the structural and vascular characteristics of the primary lesions (Fig. 63) [23]. Similarly, research of intralesional *calcifications*, typical expression of classic neoplasms – osteosarcomas, chondrosarcomas, as well as thyroidal, ovarian, and gastrointestinal carcinomas – may be extremely helpful in the diagnosis of nodal involvement [23, 26].

As mentioned previously, structural analysis of the metastatic lymph node may offer valuable prognostic information at follow-up [90]. In selected tumors, as with non-seminomatous germ cell tumors of the testes, a favorable response to chemotherapy is marked by a "cystic" transformation of the retroperitoneal lymph-

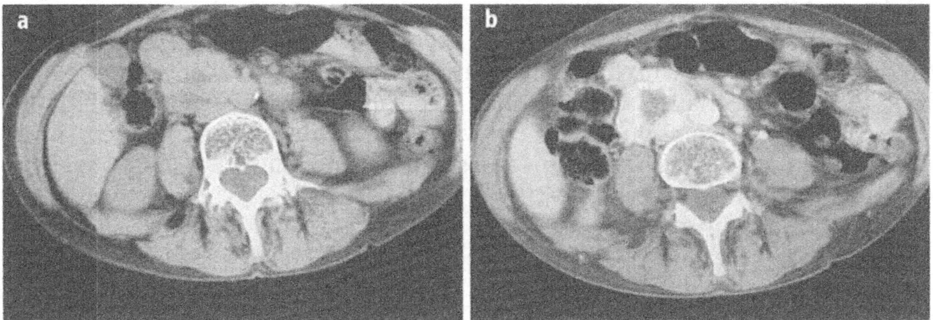

Fig. 63. Hypervascular metastasis to retroperitoneal lymph nodes, from a *colonic leiomyosarcoma*, **a** at basseline scanning and **b** after intravenous administration of contrast medium

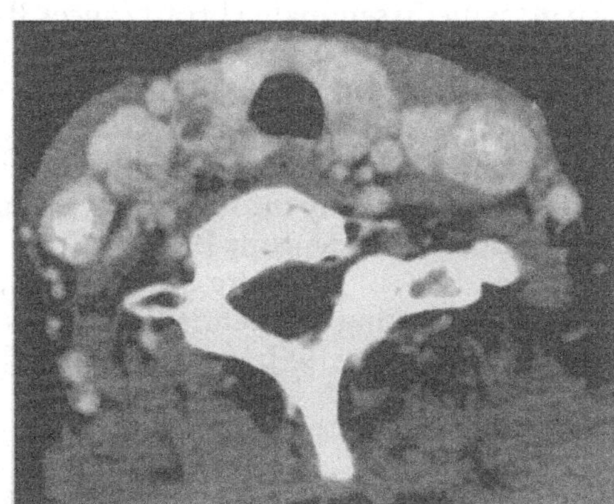

Fig. 64. Lymph node metastases with intralesional calcifications and synchronous multifocal involvement of the thyroid gland, secondary to a *mucoid adenocarcinoma of the stomach*

adenopathy, occasionally without a significant reduction in size or even in the presence of mild increase in volume (Fig. 17) [92]. The cystic involution represents the hallmark of the cellular differentiation toward more mature elements deprived of malignant potential. However, careful research of nodule or even marginal solid enhancing components is mandated in this context, since they often signify the presence of residual biologically active disease [92].

■ Rare Sites of Metastases

During the past decade detection of metastases in less than classic locations has become a statistically significant event. This is probably due to the systematic follow-up of neoplastic patients, as well as to the increased survival seen with some primary malignancies [29]. We also believe that the modern, more aggressive therapeutic protocols employed may to some extent change the biologic behavior of some tumors, maybe by selecting neoplastic subpopulations possessing elective tropism for their metastatic diffusion [93]. The marked genotypical and phenotypical instability of proliferating tumoral cells is a widely accepted notion [2]. These aspects may justify the apparently atypical relapse of disease taking place with secondary tumors in unusual locations, often without other synchronous lesions [23]. Additionally, chemotherapy may cause partial or total remission of disease for a variable length of time. But when disease does recur, it may do so in a violent fashion, thus involving organs and structures normally not interested by the majority of metastatic processes [93].

Diencephalon

Metastases to the hypothalamus–pituitary axis are frequently found at autopsy, generally in patients with widely metastatic disease [20]. Pituitary metastases represent the vast majority of these lesions and are found in 1–2% of random autopsy studies. Their incidence may, however, rise to 36% in selected series of patients with disseminated breast cancer. Breast, lung, and renal cancer are the most frequently encountered neoplasms [94, 95].

Over 80% of cases involve the posterior segment of the pituitary gland, probably because of its systemic arterial vascularization favoring the implant of neoplastic emboli (superior pituitary arteries). The anterior portion of the gland, which receives its blood supply through the hypothalamus–pituitary portal system, is rarely a site of metastatic deposits [94].

Only 6–10% of these are symptomatic, generally in the form of diabetes insipidus, thus allowing differentiation from primary adenomas which never cause this clinical abnormality [95]. Less frequently, clinical signs of insufficiency of the anter-

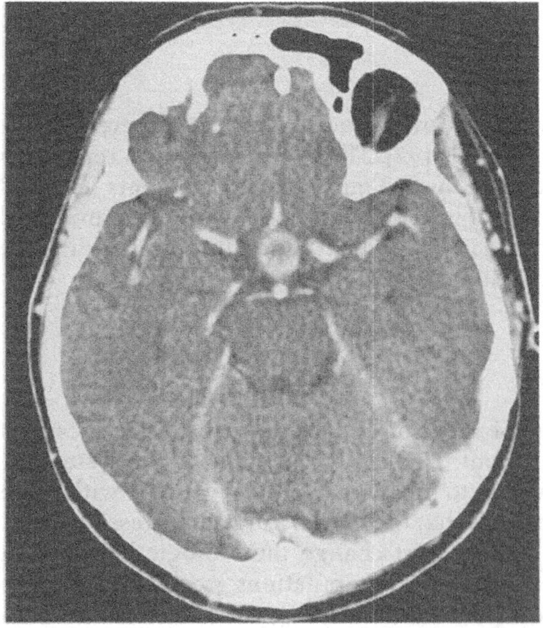

Fig. 65. Pituitary metastasis from breast carcinoma

ior gland and visual impairment may mark the clinical appearance of pituitary metastases [95].Their clinical onset and evolution is rapid, marked by the combination of gland dysfunction and cranial nerve impairment. The venous drainage from the pituitary into the cavernous sinus, which hosts the III, IV, V, and VI cranial nerves, easily accounts for the rapid neoplastic spread to these structures and relative symptoms [7].

The statistically older age, the faster onset and development of symptoms, and the positive history for oncologic disease are the most reliable differential clues against the more common adenomas, which may mimic their imaging features. Additionally, the virtually constant extrasellar extension, the disproportionate soft tissue mass with a relative paucity of bony destruction of the floor of the sella, and the synchronous involvement of the cavernous sinus with occasional leptomeningeal diffusion, are other helpful clues in the diagnosis of intrasellar metastases [94].

Computed tomography normally demonstrates lesions in the suprasellar space, with or without an intrasellar component, hypodense, with contrast enhancement (Fig. 65), often extending into the cavernous sinus and with frequent synchronous intra-axial metastases [95].

Head and Neck Region

The incidence of metastatic lesions to the head and neck region is low: Only 1% of cervico-facial neoplasms originate from primaries located below the clavicular plane [7]. The vast majority of these lesions predominately involve the *lymph nodes*, and bronchogenic, renal, breast, and gastrointestinal tract malignancies are the most frequently found histologic types [1].

The exceedingly rare extranodal locations may involve by perineural diffusion the *nervous trunks* or may invade the *paranasal sinuses* and the *nasal fossae*; these are primarily due to breast, renal, and lung cancer, and, less frequently, prostatic and cutaneous neoplasms. Their clinical appearance is non-specific as a rule, with the only exception represented by metastases due to renal cell carcinomas which often present with epistaxis [7].

In cases of distant diffusion along the preformed paths of nervous bundles, CT can demonstrate the presence of pathologic tissue obliterating the fat planes, eroding and enlarging the osseous canals and foramina, with possible secondary involvement of loco-regional anatomic crossways, such as the Meckel's cave, the pterygo-palatine fossa, the cavernous sinus, or the tympanic cave, depending on the site of origin of the neoplastic lesion. The neural invasion may in turn result in atrophy of the corresponding muscle groups. In select cases direct visualization of soft tissue cords along the course of the nerve may be possible [19, 21, 96–98] (Fig. 66). When involving the paranasal sinuses and the nasal fossae, tumoral lesions exhibit an infiltrating appearance at CT with soft tissue density and minimal contrast enhancement. The exception is again represented by metastases from renal cell carcinomas which are frequently associated with a mucocele and lytic changes of the adjacent facial skeleton (Fig. 67). The multifocal nature of these lesions is the main character which may lead to the suspicion of metastatic disease.

Orbital metastases have an incidence ranging between 3 and 12% [99]. They appear and behave differently in the pediatric and adult populations. They are more

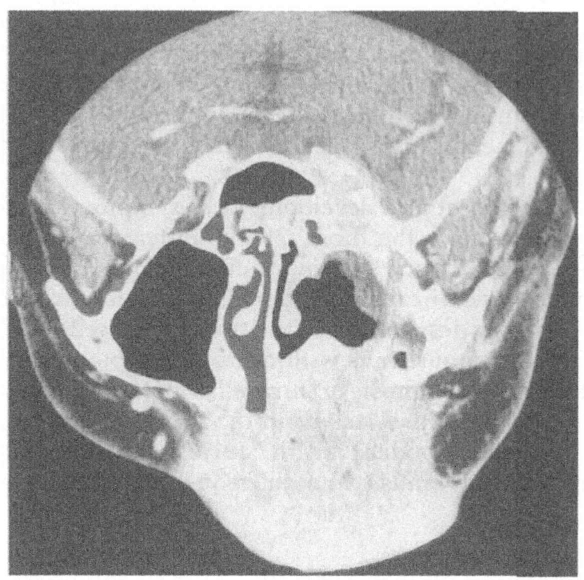

Fig. 66. Perineural diffusion along the left pterygoid canal and inferior orbital foramen from a *squamous cell carcinoma of the hard palate and alveolar ridge.* (Courtesy of S. Horowitz M. D., Loyola University Medical Center, Maywood, Ill.)

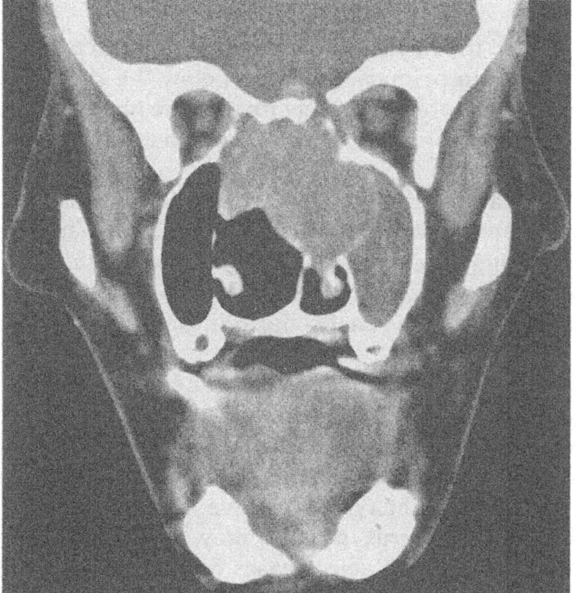

Fig. 67. Voluminous mass from *breast carcinoma*, infiltrating the left nasal fossa, eroding the medial wall of the orbit and extending into the ethmoid bone, causing secondary mucocele

often retrobulbar in the child, when they are generally due to neuroblastomas, Ewing's sarcomas, and leukemic infiltrations. In the adult population 90% of them are primarily ocular and more than half of these are secondary to breast (Fig. 68) and bronchogenic carcinomas [99]. Prostate cancer metastasizes mainly to the skeleton, with osteoslerotic localizations in the greater wing of the sphenoid which may then bulge into the orbit itself [100]. The clinical picture of a rapid onset of proptosis and ophthalmoplegia are analogous to that seen with inflammatory

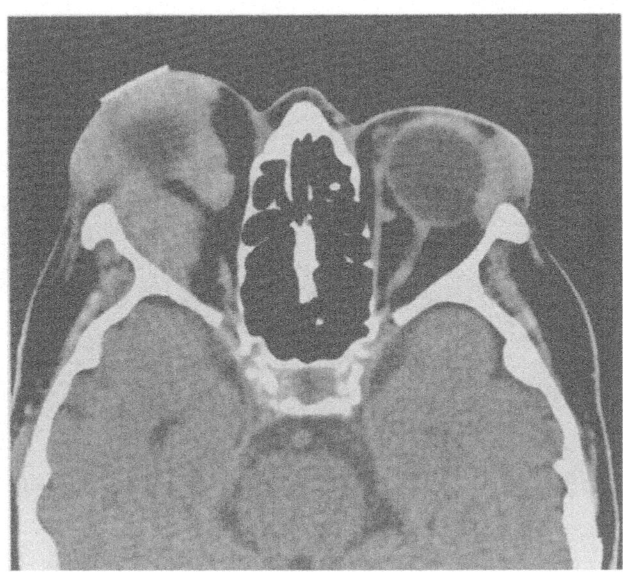

Fig. 68. Diffuse orbital metastatization from *breast carcinoma*, with both intra- and extraconal lesions

pseudotumor of the orbit, the main differential diagnostic entity; the latter, however, does not cause osseous destruction. The *uvea* and the *posterior portion of the ocular globe* are the most frequently involved sites, and the diffusion likely takes place through the posterior ciliary arteries, thereby leading to intraconal masses. Their CT appearance is characterized again by lesions with soft tissue density with variable contrast enhancement, which may infiltrate the ocular bulb and/or the surrounding oculomotor striated muscles to a variable degree [100].

Finally, extraconal lesions may extend to infiltrate the lachrymal gland, the adjacent adipose tissue, or the extraocular muscles. These lesions may appear as focal thickenings or small masses with irregular contours, heterogeneous density, with occasional extension to and destruction of the osseous orbital walls, or the extraconal tissues [99].

Thyroid and salivary glands are the other unusual sites of metastatic involvement in the head and neck region, and most other structures (pharynx, larynx, tongue, etc.) are only exceptionally invaded by metastatic lesions.

Thyroid metastases are only rarely suspected clinically. The most important clinical series report an incidence ranging from 0.4% to 7.2%, with a global mean value of approximately 3% [101]. At autopsy, however, their occurrence rises dramatically, ranging from 2% to 24%. This discrepancy and wide variability may be at least partially ascribed to the different protocols of analysis employed at different institutions, where the extent of the routine microscopic examination of the gland is not standardized [102]. It is logical to assume that without a complete microscopic examination of the gland, only those lesions macroscopically apparent would be reported, and these probably account for less than 40% of the total of thyroidal metastases [102].

The tumors that most frequently metastasize to the thyroid do so via the hematogenous route, such as melanomas (39%), renal (12%), mammary (12%), and bron-

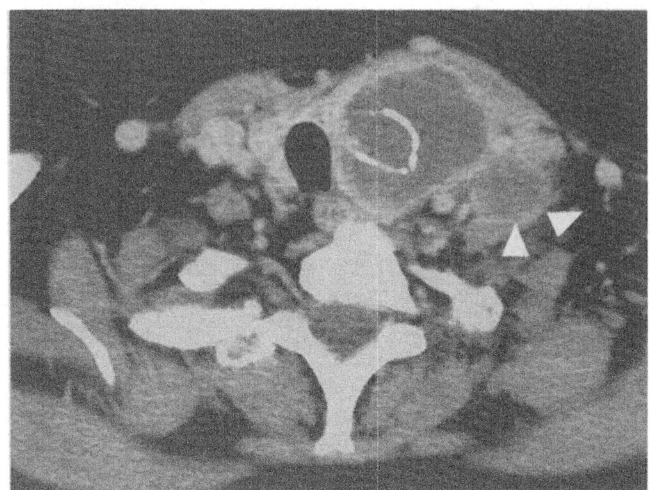

Fig. 69. Voluminous metastasis to the thyroid from *melanoma*, characterized by hypodensity due to necrosis and hemorrhage, moderate rim enhancement, and intralesional calcifications. A concurrent metastatic lymphadenopathy is demonstrated (*arrowheads*)

chogenic (11%) carcinomas. Less frequently, pancreatic and gastrointestinal tumors may also be responsible [20, 103] (Fig. 61). These are more often metachronous metastases which seem to occur after long disease-free intervals, up to 10–15 years after diagnosis of the primary tumor, especially when considering the breast and renal malignancies. Clinically, despite few scattered reports of hypo- or hyperthyroid states, the onset is marked typically by a focal or diffuse enlargement of the gland, with or without involvement of the loco-regional nodal stations, without signs of endocrine dysfunction [102]. Computed tomography may show uni- or plurifocal patterns, with a heterogeneous baseline hypodensity and moderate contrast enhancement, especially at their periphery. Hemorrhage and necrosis may also occur and are well depicted when present (Fig. 69) [102].

Salivary gland metastases are more often seen in the parotid gland, probably because of the frequent intraglandular presence of lymph nodes draining the external acoustic canal, the scalp, and portions of the face. Melanomas of the head and neck region are the most frequent source (80%), followed by squamous cell carcinomas of the proximal airway and digestive tract (mouth, tongue base, pharynx, and paranasal sinuses), breast, lung, and renal cancers.

These lesions, which often present central areas of necrosis, generally have an infiltrating appearance, without specific characters which may allow for differentiation from the markedly more common primary tumors of the previously mentioned regions. Breast and renal carcinomas may represent the exception due to their frequent marked contrast enhancement [104].

Heart

The occurrence of cardiac metastases is reported in the literature with a frequency varying between 3.4 and 5.7% [20, 65]. This low incidence has been attributed to several factors, including the continuous contractions of the heart, the high velocity of the coronary blood flow, and the metabolic peculiarities of the striated muscle cells [29, 105].

Lung, breast, as well as esophageal and pancreatic cancers, in addition to melanoma, are the primary histologic types most often responsible for this finding. Among these, melanoma is the one that shows a relatively higher tropism for the heart [7, 20, 106]. The route of diffusion has been classically considered the hematogenous one, although some recent studies have advocated a role for the cardiac lymphatics in the colonization process [7]; the latter may be a sensible explanation especially for the mammary and bronchogenic metastases in which synchronous hilar and subcarinal lymphadenopathies have a higher incidence. From these stations retrograde diffusion along the lymphatics to the cardiac district can be postulated [8, 106]. The lymphatic obstruction caused by tumor determines interstitial edema of the myocardium. The extrinsic pressure secondarily exerted upon the myofibrils may then cause the onset of cardiac failure especially in those patients with underlying coronary artery disease [105]. Cardiac metastases usually belong to a wider picture of diffuse metastatic disease; only seldom does the cardiac or pericardial involvement represent an isolated event [7].

The most frequent appearance of cardiac metastases is of typical multiple nodules of variable size, well demarcated from each other, whereas the diffuse permeative growth has been described in sarcomatous malignancies [29]. Metastatic lesions may involve the pericardium, myocardium, endocardium, valves, and coronary arteries. Alternatively, tumoral extension via the venae cavae or the pulmonary veins into the cardiac chambers may lead to large endocavitary masses capable of significant obstruction to the venous return or to the valves themselves [105]. This venous route of diffusion is typical of renal and hepatic carcinomas, as well as uterine leiomyosarcomas. Imaging detection of involvement of the right atrium may be arduous in borderline cases, but it bears significant implications for the surgical approach and therefore for the prognosis of these patients [50–51].

The CT appearance is marked by focal or diffuse mural thickenings, or by endoluminal hypodense masses (Fig. 70). Pericardial effusion represents a frequent association and is virtually always seen when in the presence of intrathoracic sites of primary origin.

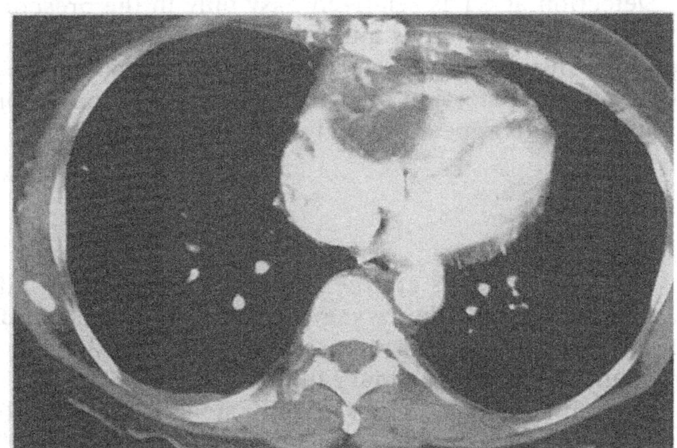

Fig. 70. Intraluminal infiltrating metastasis from *melanoma*

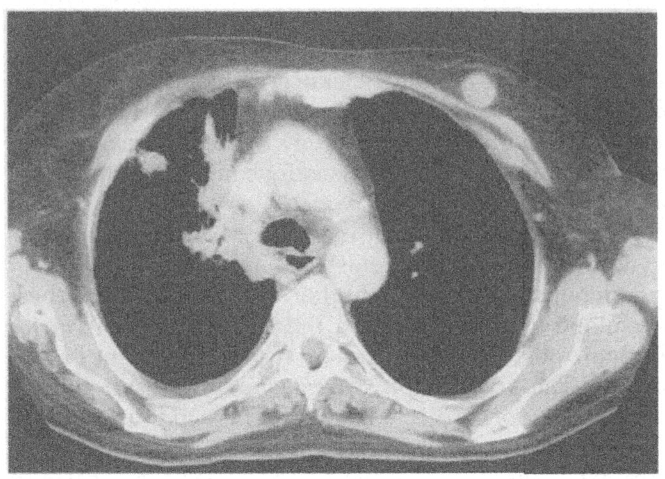

Fig. 71. Well-defined smoothly marginated nodule in the left breast, secondary to an *adenocarcinoma of the lung*

Breast

The breast is a rare location for metastatic disease. According to autopsy series, the incidence of breast metastases varies between 1.2 and 6.6% depending on whether leukemic and lymphomatous infiltrations are included [20]. They occur primarily through hematogenous spread or alternatively via the lymphatic vessels [7]. The most frequent lesion is the melanoma (22%), followed by lung cancer (18%), ovarian carcinoma (11%), and sarcomas (8%) [69]. In addition, prostate carcinoma represents a relatively frequent source of metastases to the male breast [107].

Breast metastases are most often solitary (85%), unilateral (75%), and superficial lesions, with a clear predilection for the lateral upper quadrant, without associated cutaneous changes or microcalcifications [107]. Their contours are round and regular, without peripheral spiculations related to fibrous reaction [108, 109]. Multiple bilateral and diffuse lesions are far less common and indicate a tumultuous growth [110, 111].

Detection at CT is relatively easy only in the presence of a gland with adipose involution. In such cases multiple lesions with soft tissue density, with well-defined contours may be appreciated. Alternatively, focal abnormalities with suggestion of architectural distortion of the gland and surrounding planes may be seen and are non-specific in appearance (Fig. 71) [29].

Gallbladder

The gallbladder is another rare site of secondary diffusion of malignant neoplasms, with an incidence varying from 1 to 5%, depending on the series analyzed [112]. Melanomas, lung, pancreatic, gastric, and renal carcinomas are the most frequent originating primary tumors [20, 69, 113].

The different modalities of diffusion, at least in the early stages, affect the pathologic and imaging characteristics of the lesions. The most frequent route of

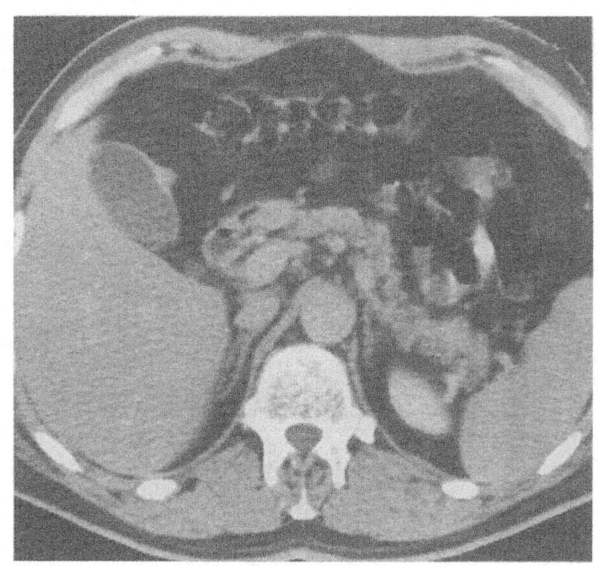

Fig. 72. Small subserosal focal thickening of the gallbladder wall due to transperitoneal diffusion from a *gastric adenocarcinoma*

metastatization is hematogenous, especially when in the presence of melanomas and pulmonary neoplasms. In such cases the CT appearance is given by multiple nodular or vegetating lesions, which may later grow to efface the entire lumen and therefore simulate a primary malignancy [7, 114]. These lesions are very well documented by cholangio-CT and appear as multiple hypodense filling defects adhering to the cholecystic wall [112].

The lymphatic diffusion is, on the other hand, more often associated with a diffuse infiltration of the cholecystic wall, which appears irregularly thickened and non-distensible, with mild contrast enhancement. When the neoplastic process finally disrupts the mucosal lining from underneath, vegetating masses may be seen within the gallbladder lumen (Fig. 72) [7, 112].

Transperitoneal colonization, by cellular migration through the peritoneal leaflets, leads to the formation of subserosal nodules, iso- or hypodense in texture [7, 112]. The subserosal lesions are typically asymptomatic and discovered incidentally at follow-up. On the other hand, metastatic lesions causing full thickness disease of the gallbladder wall or large fungating masses may occasionally be the cause of colicky pain or acute inflammatory processes.

The occasional polypoid lesions may pose problems of differential diagnosis against cholecystic primary benign and malignant tumors. The concurrent presence of cholelithiasis may be of help since it is found in approximately 80–90% of the primary carcinomas of the gallbladder. Diffusely infiltrating processes may, on the other hand, simulate chronic sclero-atrophic cholecystitis [112].

Pancreas

Pancreatic metastases are believed to be infrequent. In the literature their incidence varies between 3 and 37%, depending on whether the study was based on

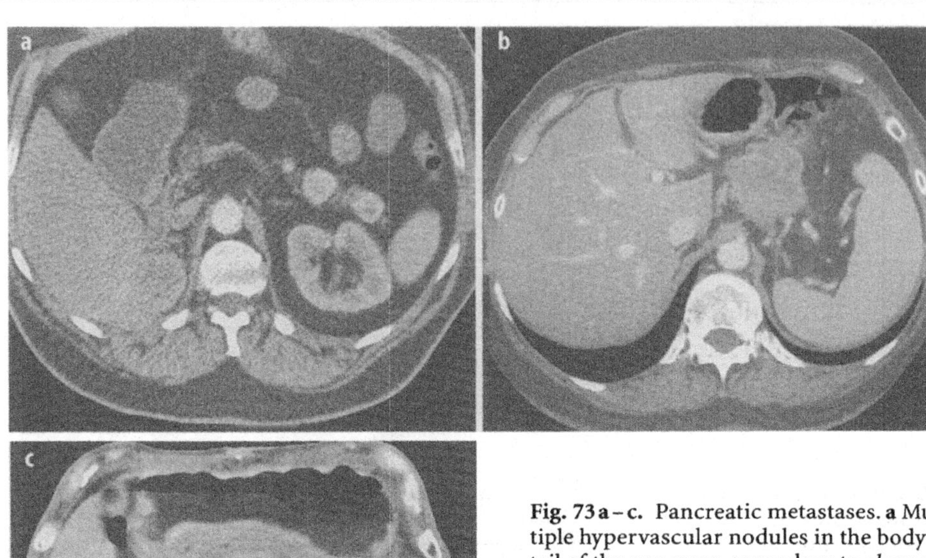

Fig. 73 a–c. Pancreatic metastases. **a** Multiple hypervascular nodules in the body and tail of the pancreas, secondary to *clear cell carcinoma of the kidney*. **b** Large heterogeneous lesions of the pancreatic isthmus, from a *colonic carcinoma*, causing gross focal abnormality of the glandular contour. **c** Diffuse lymphangitic infiltration of the pancreatic parenchyma, from a *sigmoid adenocarcinoma*, with marked secondary desmoplastic reaction

random autopsy series or relative to patients affected by highly metastasizing tumors, such as melanoma, lung or breast cancer [20, 115]. Their incidence in vivo is, however, underestimated, given the paucity of both clinical symptoms (jaundice, acute pancreatitis) and specific pancreatic laboratory values (serum and urinary amylase) [93]. In addition to the aforementioned malignancies renal, gastric and colic cancers are among the most frequently responsible primary tumors [116].

The process takes place most typically through the hematogenous route, although lymphatic diffusion is not infrequent, often by retrograde diffusion from loco-regional lymphadenopathies, or through the peritoneum [7, 115].

An important complication along the course of a pancreatic secondary tumor is represented by acute pancreatitis, which is occasionally of the necrotic–hemorrhagic type. The two most probable mechanisms are a neoplastic obstruction of Wirsung's duct and an acute tumoral cellular lysis secondary to chemotherapy [93, 117, 118].

The tomodensitometric appearance of pancreatic metastases is classified according to three main patterns (Fig. 73):

1. The most typical pattern is represented by multiple nodules which occasionally coalesce in larger masses (Fig. 12). The CT density of these neoplastic foci is variable and usually related to the histologic type of the originating primary tumor. However, they appear most often hypodense; contrast enhancement is

appreciable in the early arterial phase only in those tumors secondary to hyper-vascular primary tumors [93, 119].

2. The second aspect is marked by the presence of a solitary mass which causes alteration of the gland contour; these often present with a heterogeneous structure secondary to necrotic or degenerative phenomena [120]. Their epicenter accounts for the onset of symptoms and CT signs. If, for example, it is located in the head, the mass determines neoplastic obstruction of the common biliary duct, with jaundice, and/or of Wirsung's duct, with atrophy of the pancreatic body and tail, and beading of Wirsung's duct itself. In this subgroup of patients elevated amylasemia is a frequent finding, secondary to acinar destruction [93, 117].

3. The last pattern, lymphangitic in appearance, is marked by a diffuse involvement of the gland, which in later stages appears enlarged and homogeneously hypodense [93]. Such aspects are seen most often with breast and lung cancers and are characterized by a permeative growth of neoplastic cords along the interlobular septa which finally causes destruction of the pancreatic lobules. This appearance may be difficult to differentiate from a lymphomatous localization, especially in the presence of local lymphonodal involvement [93].

The CT appearance of the pancreas may be entirely normal in the early phases, when small metastases do not alter the organ contour or cause a conspicuous attenuation gradient. Thin collimation or dynamic helical scanning may, however, ameliorate sensitivity [115].

Lymphomas and primary adenocarcinomas of the pancreas are the main entities of the differential diagnosis, especially in light of the possibility of a second primary neoplasm in patients with a known malignancy [93]. Venous stasis, secondary to nodal compression of the splenic vein, may also cause increase in gland size and therefore simulate a metastatic involvement of the third type [93].

Spleen

Splenic metastases are found in approximately 7–10% of patients who died because of neoplastic disease [20, 29, 121, 122]. They are generally secondary to hematogenous diffusion through the splenic artery. However, a retrograde colonization via the splenic vein can be caused by pancreatic tumors or, in the presence of portal obstruction or hypertension, by gastrointestinal malignancies [7]. Much less common are the lymphatic and transperitoneal routes of involvement [7, 121, 122].

Breast, bronchogenic, ovarian, and gastric carcinomas, as well as melanomas, pancreatic and colon adenocarcinomas, and hepatocellular carcinomas are the most frequent primary tumors metastasizing to the spleen [20, 121, 122], especially in the setting of generalized neoplastic disease.

Macroscopically, the lesions may exhibit nodular morphology, solitary or multiple, or may appear as a diffuse infiltrative process. Their appearance at CT is characterized typically by round hypodense nodules, well defined when small, and ill defined if larger. An occasional peripheral rim of contrast enhancement and central necrotic phenomena may also be detected [29]. Cystic and pseudo-cystic features are not rare, especially with ovarian carcinomas or necrotizing lesions such as melano-

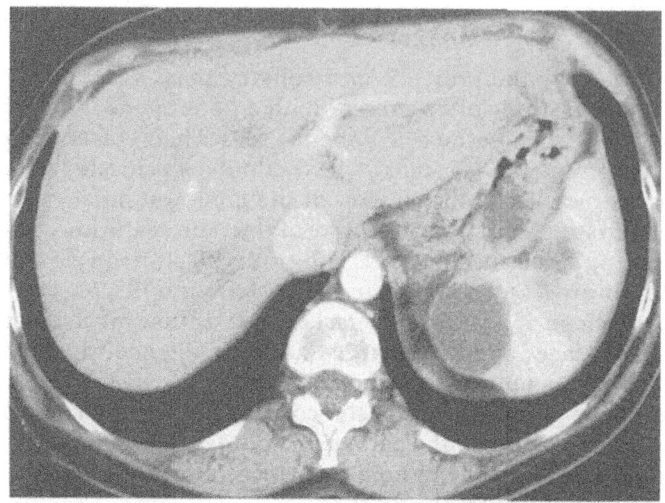

Fig. 74. Cystic splenic metastasis originating from a *serious cystadeno-carcinoma of the ovary*

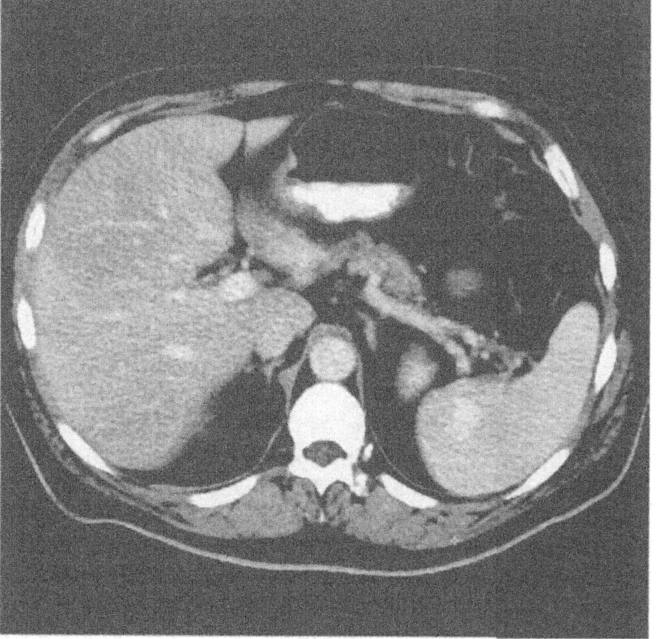

Fig. 75. Hypervascular splenic metastasis from *carcinoid of the small bowel*

mas. These cystic structures, when of small dimensions, may be confused with primary cysts or hemangiomas of the spleen which, along with inflammatory or granulomatous processes, represent the primary differential diagnostic possibilities (Fig. 74) [29]. Detection of hyperdense masses (Fig. 75) is rare and normally related to metastases from classically hyperdense primary tumors. Solitary masses normally do not display any specific characteristic to allow reliable differentiation from other primary splenic neoplasms such as lymphomas and angiosarcomas [123].

Gastrointestinal System

Metastatic localizations to the gastrointestinal system are an infrequent occurrence and generally represent metachronous lesions, frequently occurring after a long time from the diagnosis of the primary lesion [124]. Their diagnosis is often delayed due to the relative lack of specificity of symptoms. Differential diagnosis toward benign and malignant primary tumors, as well as against radiation changes, is often problematic [125].

There is a fundamental relation between the route of metastatic colonization and the macroscopic appearance of these metastases. Their pattern may preferentially be fungating, nodular intramural, infiltrating or subserosal, depending on the location of the lesions and the histologic type involved [124].

In order to accurately detect and possibly characterize metastases to the gastrointestinal tract, rigorous and sophisticated techniques must be employed during the CT examination. Parameters such as the collimation thickness, window of display, scanning time, intravenous contrast medium administration rate, and optimal distention and opacification of the visceral lumen all play valuable roles. As already proposed by some authors [126], we believe that plain water is an optimal contrast medium to obtain distention of the stomach and colon, whereas iodinated media or diluted barium sulfate are ideal to opacify the esophagus and small bowel.

Esophagus

The esophagus is the rarest site of localization along the alimentary tract, with a frequency varying between 0.6 and 3% [20, 29, 127]. Colonization occurs mostly through the lymphatics [14]. Lung and breast cancer are the most frequently encountered primary sources. Thyroidal and gastric carcinomas are seen less often [7, 124, 127, 128]. Dysphagia, often with sudden onset, is a virtually always present symptom [125].

Secondarily to the lymphatic spread, the lesions are mostly infiltrating and/or subserosal, with a predilection for the middle third of the viscus, where there is the largest number of lymphatic connections [124]. At CT there is irregular thickening of the wall, often associated with other signs of mediastinal disease such as lymphadenopathy, carcinomatosis and fibrosis [29] (Fig. 76). Transdiaphragmatic diffusion, seen especially with tumors of the stomach or of the lung bases, alternatively cause annular strictures of the lower esophageal third [127].

Blood-borne metastases are rare and virtually always secondary to melanomas, typically causing multiple fungating or intramural masses [69]. Ulceration is a less frequent complication in this location than what is seen in the gastric and intestinal districts [29, 125].

The differential diagnosis includes post-radiation esophagitis, seen primarily in patients treated for breast carcinomas, and, less frequently, peptic esophagitis, benign and malignant primary tumors of the esophagus [124].

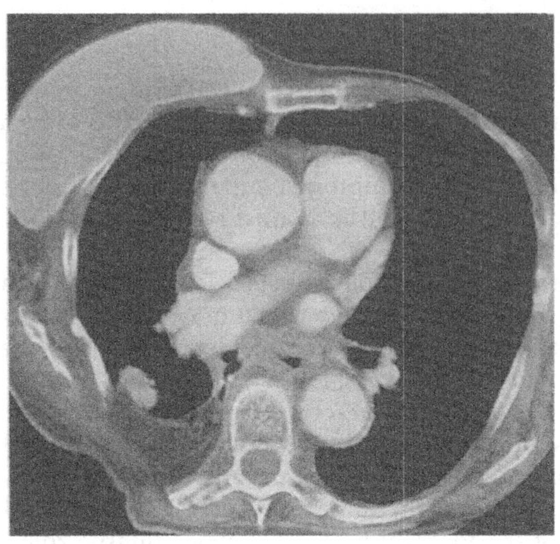

Fig. 76. Irregular parietal metastatic thickening of the thoracic esophagus in patient with prior mastectomy for *breast carcinoma*. The patient also exhibits simultaneous local recurrence of disease after right lower lobectomy for pulmonary adenocarcinoma

Stomach

Random autopsy series show a 0.7% incidence of gastric metastases, which rise to 8–26% in selected oncologic series [20, 124]. Melanomas as well as breast and bronchogenic carcinomas are the main primary sources, followed, less commonly, by hepatocellular carcinomas, head and neck cancers, and chorioncarcinomas [7, 125, 129].

Diffuse abdominal discomfort and/or pain, anorexia, dysphagia, nausea, and vomiting represent common albeit non-specific symptoms. Ulcerated and necrotic masses eroding through the mucosa may result in gastrointestinal bleeding which may either be apparent through hematemesis or sideropenic anemia [124, 129].

Metastatic diffusion to the stomach occurs most frequently through the hematogenous route [7], typically with melanomas and lung cancers. These result in multiple submucosal lesions, which may grow toward the lumen or the subserosal surface [125]. Mucosal involvement may cause either elevated lesions with central depression due to ulcerative necrosis (bull's-eye lesions) or frankly fungating intraluminal masses [129].

A lymphangitic pattern, typical of breast carcinomas, determines, on the other hand, a diffuse parietal infiltration, with a "pseudolinitis plastica" appearance [7, 20]. The tumor, originally submucosal in location, later extends to the entire thickness of the gastric wall, probably also due to the massive neoplastic embolization of the capillary and lymphatic network [7, 29]. The late appearance at CT is that of a rigid tubular viscus, with multiple spicules due to omental and peritoneal tractions [124]. Focal stenoses, especially in the antral segment, are another non infrequent possible appearance [130].

Direct transperitoneal extension is instead unusual and takes place by diffusion through a ligamentous attachment of the mesenterium or the gastro-colic ligament, as in carcinomas of the transverse and descending colon. Permeation of the lymphatic routes, as in esophageal cancers and tumors of the lower pulmonary lobes,

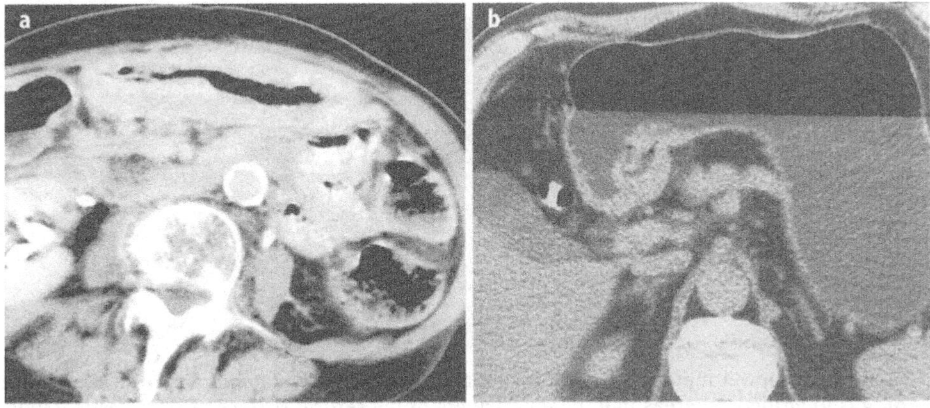

Fig. 77 a, b. Gastric metastases. **a** "Pseudolinitis plastica" from *breast carcinoma*, with mildly hypodense parietal thickening of the viscus which appears diffusely rigid and non-distensible. **b** Secondary polypoid lesion of the posterior antrum with central ulcerative necrosis, from a *retroperitoneal leiomyosarcoma*

rarely allows transdiaphragmatic extension with prevalent involvement of the gastric fundus and proximal body [7, 29, 79]. Again the late appearance is that of subserosal nodules or infiltrating plaques [124].

The pseudolinitis plastica is characterized at CT by diffuse and hypodense infiltrations involving the majority of the viscus and exhibiting scarce contrast enhancement; the tumor may occasionally show signs of transerosal extension [130, 131]. Otherwise, solitary or multiple nodular or vegetating lesions may, on the other hand, be detected, at times limited to focal non-specific thickenings of the wall, all mimicking primary adenocarcinoma of the stomach [131, 132] (Fig. 77).

The differential diagnosis of the lymphangitic form is against lymphoma, primary gastric cancer, and Kaposi's sarcoma [29, 75]. Multiple nodular patterns may mimic carcinoids, polyps, and again, lymphomas and Kaposi's sarcomas [75, 124, 132], whereas solitary vegetating lesions may resemble mesenchymal tumors (leiomyomas and neurofibromas), carcinoids, ectopic pancreatomas, adenocarcinomas, and less frequently, primary lymphomas [29, 75, 129, 131, 132].

Small Bowel

Despite difficult assessment of the primary or secondary origin of an intestinal lesion, neoplasms from ovaries, uterus, or sigmoid are statistically the most frequent sources of secondary intestinal lesions [7, 20, 125]. Direct transperitoneal extension, from a non-contiguous pelvic primary tumor, takes place via fasciae and mesenteric attachments and is typical of neoplasms with highly malignant and destructive potential [79, 124, 125]. Intestinal involvement secondary to peritoneal carcinomatosis is very common especially in ovarian carcinomas [17].

Lymphatic diffusion is rare and generally secondary to distant tumors, probably by retrograde diffusion from metastatic lymphadenopathies and inversion of the lymphatic flow [10, 17, 80].

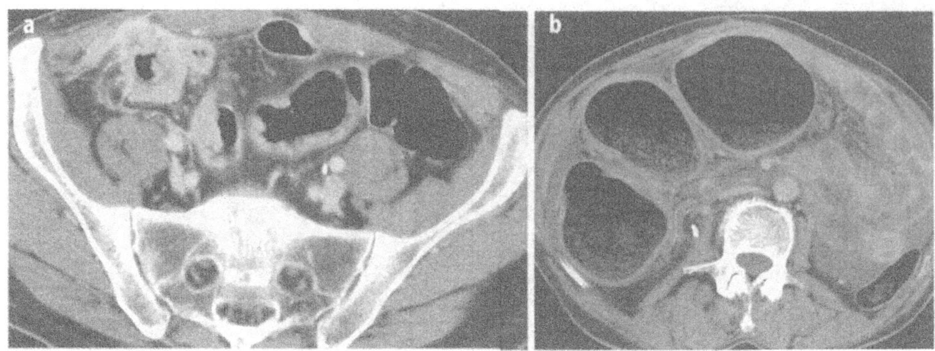

Fig. 78a, b. Small bowel metastases, both secondary to *ovarian carcinomas*. In **a** diffuse parietal thickening is identified, whereas in **b** the involvement of the serosal surface of the intestinal loops is marked by irregular thickening of the visceral walls and secondary partial obstruction

Hematogenous diffusion is relatively frequent. Melanomas are responsible for approximately one third of these blood-borne metastases [7, 45, 69, 124], followed by breast, lung, colon, and kidney carcinomas [20, 124, 133].

Metastatic lesions, which initially originate within the submucosal layer of the viscus, later tend to expand toward the mucosal plane with vegetating and ulcerated masses [124]. The predominantly endoluminal growth accounts for the relatively high incidence of intussusception [124, 134]. Hemorrhage is also a frequent complication, especially with metastatic melanomas and renal cell carcinomas [69, 135]. Clinically, the most frequent finding is chronic bleeding [125]. When in the presence of large masses, intussusception or bowel occlusion are typical consequences [125], whereas bowel wall perforation is relatively rare [136].

Computed tomography accurately depicts the pathologic findings (Fig. 78): *intraluminal fungating* lesions, or non-descript soft tissue density filling defects, easily delineated when the viscus is adequately distended and opacified [29, 124]; an *ulcerated appearance* with the classic appearance of "plus in minus," with occasional clear cavitations [125, 137], and bull's-eye or target appearance; foci of *parietal thickening*, which may be segmental, causing alternating areas of stenoses and dilatations (typically seen with breast cancer), or diffusely involving a relatively long tract of small bowel which appears fixed, with a rigid and often sharply angulated course of the terminal ileal loops secondary to invasion and "freezing" of the mesentery [15, 125, 135]; *subserosal localizations* manifesting as marginal surface irregularities or as large, predominately extrinsic masses associated with other signs of peritoneal carcinomatosis (ascites), involvement of the mesentery, and other peritoneal surfaces, as well as mesenteric lymphadenopathies [77, 124].

The main differential diagnostic challenges are represented at such level by local primary neoplasms primarily, lymphomas. Post-radiation changes, in patients treated for abdominal or pelvic neoplasms, and abdominal endometriosis, may also be difficult to distinguish [15, 29, 75]. The absence of desmoplastic reaction effacing the mesenteric adipose tissue may help in differentiating hematogenous metastases from intestinal carcinoids or scirrhous carcinomas [69, 124, 137].

Colon and Rectum

The incidence of metastases in colon and rectum is reportedly approximately 1 % [20]. The most frequent targets are the cecum and the transverse colon, with pelvic neoplasms being the prime etiologies, particularly prostate and ovarian cancer [124].

Tumoral diffusion, through the omentum and other peritoneal folds, probably represents the main pattern of metastatic colonization to the colon [1, 7]. This process allows gastric and pancreatic cancers to extend to the transverse colon through the gastrocolic ligament and the transverse mesocolon, renal cell carcinomas to spread to the descending colon, and pelvic malignancies to metastasize to the transverse colon [10, 15, 80, 138]. Their appearance is most often infiltrating with or without macroscopic extension to the subserosal surface [124].

Transperitoneal diffusion takes place frequently in the sigmoid colon, a classic target for metastases originating from ovarian carcinomas [7, 124, 125]. Blood-borne metastases appear less frequently and tend to show the same etiologies and the same patterns of growth as seen in the small bowel [29, 124].

Clinically, colonic metastases may have an insidious and non-specific manifestation, with pain being the most frequent symptom, especially in the presence of extensive peritoneal involvement [124]. Otherwise, the rarity of acute obstruction and of symptoms often delays clinical suspicion of neoplastic invasion.

At CT their appearance is again characterized by fungating masses, parietal thickenings of variable extent, or subserosal nodules as already described in the small bowel (Fig. 79) [15, 29, 124].

Infiltration of the sigmoid walls from peritoneal neoplasms of ovarian origin may frequently appear indistinguishable from an ovarian primary that has gained foot onto the mesosigma and the sigmoid itself by direct continuity [77]. Pseudo-tumoral inflammatory masses from acute diverticular disease or radiation-induced fibrosis are additional entities to be considered in the differential diagnosis [124].

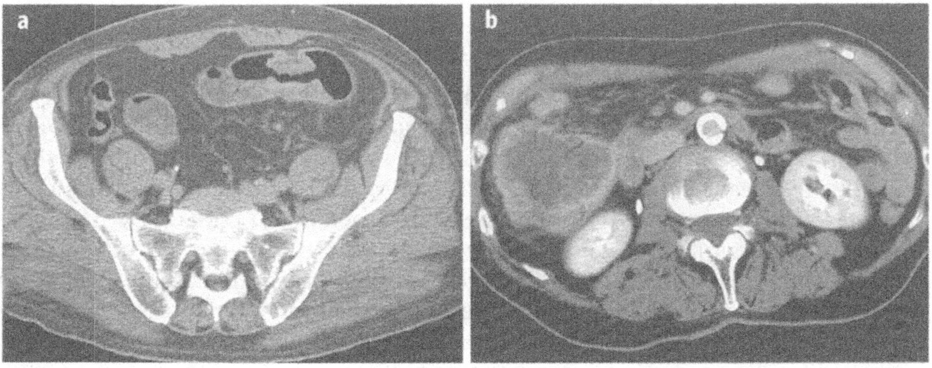

Fig. 79. Colonic metastases from *melanomas*, with **a** a polypoid appearance and **b** diffuse and irregular mural thickening and transmural extension through the serosa into adjacent planes

Kidney

The finding of renal secondary neoplastic involvement is a frequent occurrence at autopsy, ranging from 2% to 20% depending on the sources and the selection of the cases [20, 139]. In decreasing order of frequency, the most common sites of origin of primary malignancies are the lung, breast, stomach, pancreas, colon, kidney, and esophagus [7, 20, 139]. Melanomas, which metastasize to the kidney in up to 37% of cases, making this organ one of its most important targets, accounts for only 2% of renal secondary tumors diagnosed at autopsy, due to the relative low incidence of melanomas among neoplasms [140].

The typical route of diffusion is generally hematogenous, resulting in preferential cortical involvement [7]. On the other hand, the lymphatics have been advocated as the most probable route of spread, when in the presence of lesions extending to the perirenal spaces. The intercostal, juxta-vertebral, and para-aortic lymph nodes would represent the intermediate stations [141].

Typically, renal metastases appear as multiple, bilateral lesions with nodules smaller than 2 cm [140]. However, not infrequently, solitary large lesions are encountered, especially with secondary large bowel malignancies [29].

Renal metastases are often associated with secondary involvement of other organs, thus signifying a generalized disease. Depending on the causative primary tumors, liver, lungs, adrenal glands, and lymph nodes are the most frequently identified locations of synchronous invasion [20, 139].

In the majority of cases, renal metastases are asymptomatic. These patients report only minor and vague complaints, such as lumbar pain or discomfort. Microhematuria is occasional and proteinuria is extraordinary [140].

Renal metastases demonstrate an ample range of morphostructural appearances (Figs. 80, 81):

1. Multiple bilateral hypodense lesions, more often small (5–15 mm), with only mild contrast enhancement [139].
2. Solitary, generally voluminous masses with colliquative necrosis giving fluid central densities and ill-defined contours, a pattern often detected in secondary colonic carcinomas [139].
3. Single solid lesions, of variable size, with well-defined and grossly regular contours, homogeneously iso- or, rarely, hyperdense at baseline, and predominantly hypovascular after contrast medium administration [29].
4. Lesions with involvement of the peri-renal space, often seen as bulging nodules extending into, and effacing, the perirenal space, or, less frequently, as thin curvilinear streaks infiltrating the perirenal space. Nodular thickenings of the renal fascia are occasionally seen in metastatic melanoma [140, 141].
5. Hemorrhagic lesions are, as previously stated, typical of hypervascular primary tumors which may therefore demonstrate mild contrast enhancement. Depending on the age of the hemorrhage, the tomodensitometric features may range from an inhomogeneously hyperdense texture at baseline, to a *hematocrit level*, to a frankly *pseudo-cystic*-appearing mass [139].
6. Masses with calcification, which may appear as coarse central foci, multiple nodules generally associated to necrotic phenomena, or as peripheral egg-shell-like rims. The primary tumors are osteosarcoma, chondrosarcoma, and mucinous or papillary carcinomas [26, 140].

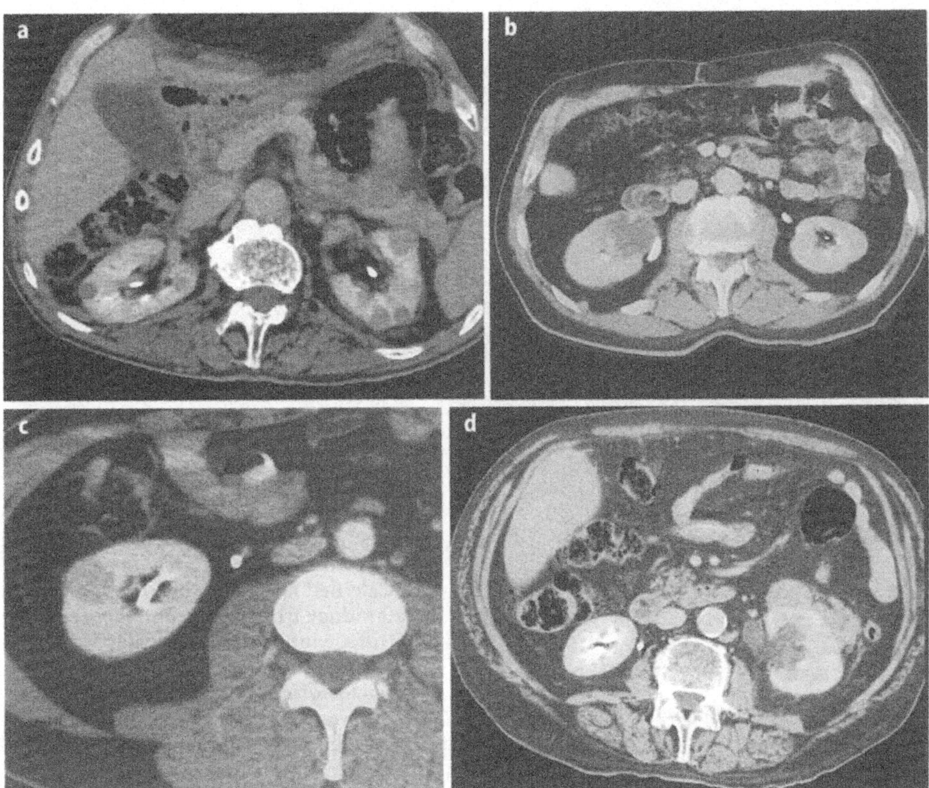

Fig. 80a–d. Renal metastases. a Multiple bilateral hypodense nodules from *pulmonary adeno-carcinoma*. b Solitary mass of the right kidney, with necrotic density, from a *carcinoma of the ileo-cecal valve*. c Mildly heterogeneous hypodense nodule of the right kidney in a patient with prior left nephrectomy for *clear cell adenocarcinoma*. d Multiple nodules of the perirenal space from a *bronchogenic carcinoma*

7. Diffusely infiltrating lesions, with a "lymphangitic appearance," massively involving the kidney, which appears globally enlarged and hypodense [29, 140].

The differential diagnosis includes cysts and frank cortical infarcts (not infrequent during paraneoplastic coagulopathies) in the presence of multiple small and bilateral lesions [29]. Large bilateral nodules may resemble lymphomas or synchronous renal cell carcinomas. Solitary masses may be confused with primary benign (oncocytoma, angiomyolipoma with a prevalent myoid component, leiomyoma) and malignant (carcinomas, sarcomas, lymphomas) tumors [75, 140]. Inflammatory/infectious processes (during acute pancreatitis and other retroperitoneal inflammations), hemorrhagic complications of traumatic or systemic processes, lymphomas, and venous or lymphatic collaterals may all resemble a secondary neoplastic colonization of the perirenal and pararenal spaces [75, 139, 141]. Amorphous intralesional components may also be seen with primary renal cell carcinomas or in cysts with calcified walls [140].

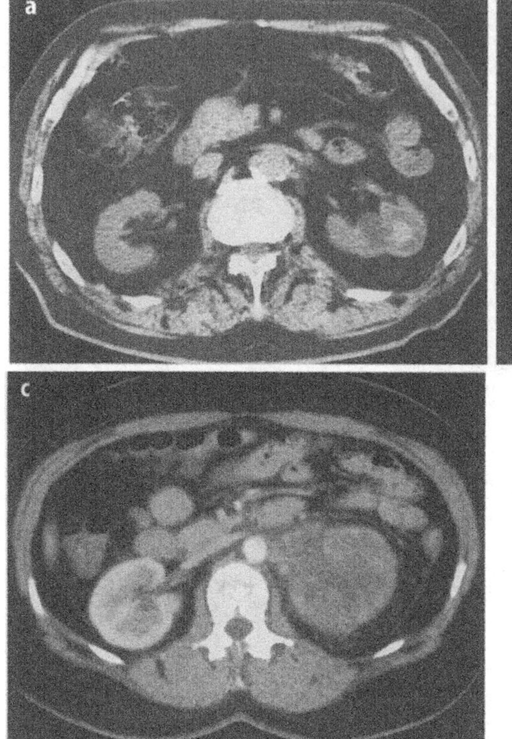

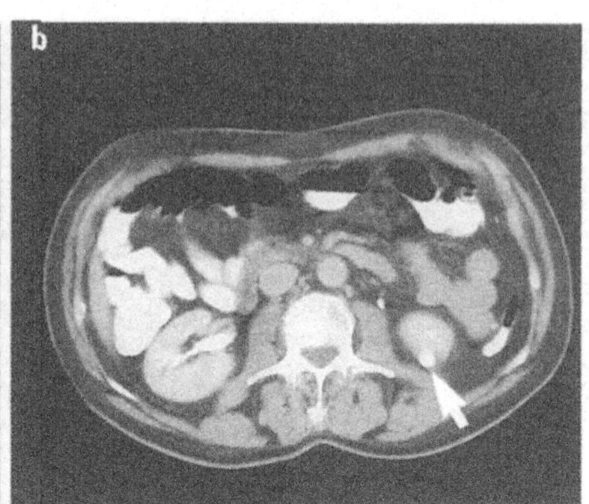

Fig. 81 a – c. Renal metastases. **a** Hemorrhagic mass of the left kidney with heterogeneous hyperdensity, representing a metastasis from a *leiomyosarcoma of the thigh*. **b** Calcified nodule of the lower pole of the left kidney from an *osteosarcoma (arrow)*. **c** Diffuse infiltration of the left kidney, lymphangitic in appearance, secondary to *metastatic pancreatic carcinoma*. The kidney appears globally infiltrated and increased in volume, with a predominantly hypodense structure

Ureter and Bladder

Ureteral metastases are very rare and are generally detected at autopsy as part of disseminated metastatic disease [20]. Breast carcinoma (especially of the lobular subtype), colon cancer, and melanomas are the most frequent causative primary tumors [7, 29, 142].

They appear at CT as segmental mural thickenings, with a secondary hydroureteronephrosis. Secondary urinomas have also been described [29, 142].

Bladder metastases, on the other hand, are believed to arise from lymphatic spread of intrapelvic malignancies, especially from the colon–rectum and prostate gland [7, 20, 80]. They generally exhibit an infiltrating pattern of growth, not discernible from primary malignancies when in advanced stage (Fig. 82). Disseminated forms, with vegetating intraluminal masses, are, on the other hand, often secondary to melanomas [29, 45].

Female Genital System

The *ovary* is the only organ in this system that exhibits a statistically significant incidence of secondary neoplasms, representing approximately 30 % of ovarian neoplasms [20, 143]. The correct diagnosis is often difficult to obtain, due to their

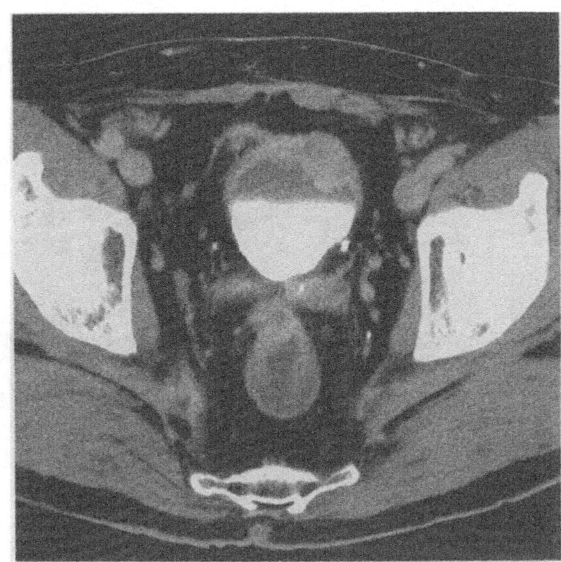

Fig. 82. Extensive metastatic colonization of the anterior wall of the bladder, from an *adenocarcinoma of the rectum*, with mixed vegetating and infiltrating features

difficult differentiation from primary neoplasms and because the presenting symptoms may often be related to the ovaries themselves before the primary lesion is clinically apparent and known [143].

The mechanism of diffusion is primarily lymphatic for pelvic neoplasms (mostly uterus), whereas hematogenous and transperitoneal diffusion have been considered as the preferential routes of colonizations for distant tumors [7].

In decreasing order of frequency the responsible primary tumors are colon, stomach, breast, pancreas, gallbladder, and bronchogenic carcinomas, as well as melanoma [7, 20, 143].

Ovarian metastases are generally bilateral, inhomogeneously solid (such as those from the stomach), cystic (from colon), or with a mixed appearance. These tumors, which exhibit variable enhancement, are often characterized by septa, papillary protrusion, as well as thickened and vascularized walls, especially when from colonic tumors [20, 144]. Lesions with foci of calcification have also been described, due to mucin-secreting neoplasms of the gastro-intestinal tract (Fig. 83) [145].

The *vagina* is the second site of metastatic occurrence in the female genital tract. The primary tumors are both genital and extragenital neoplasms [143]. Ovarian and colorectal neoplasms are the most frequently encountered primary tumors, generally extending through the pelvic lymphatic plexus. Renal cell carcinomas, after thrombosis of the left renal vein, may also cause retrograde embolization of the utero-vaginal plexus through the ovarian vein with subsequent appearance of a solitary vaginal or vulvar metastasis [1]. Computed tomography demonstrates focal lesions, more often hypodense in texture, with a non-specific appearance [29].

With the exception of the intragenital spread, metastatic localizations to the *vulva, salpinges,* and *uterus* are exceedingly rare. Selected primary tumors may occasionally synchronously diffuse to multiple viscera, with simultaneous lesions in the uterus, salpinges, and vulva [7, 143].

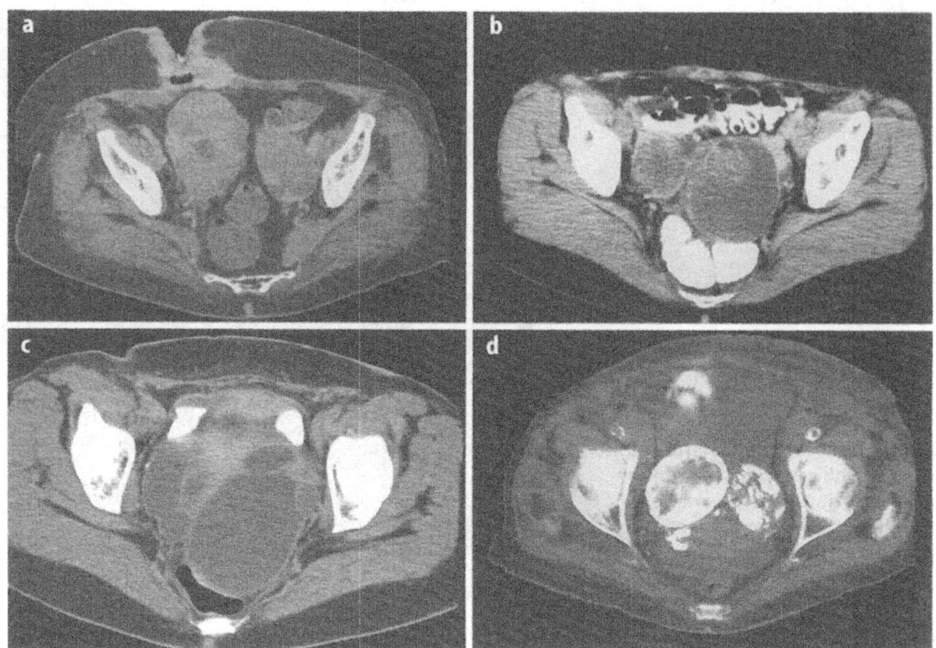

Fig. 83. Ovarian metastases from *adenocarcinoma of the colon*, solid and heterogeneous due to **a** necrosis, **b** mixed cystic and solid, **c** strictly cystic, and **d** with coarse extensive calcifications

These metastases are mostly secondary to lymphatic diffusion of colorectal malignancies which may simulate a primary tumor, especially in the presence of a solitary endometrial lesion [29, 80, 143]. Hematogenous localizations from melanomas as well as breast and lung cancer are exceptional and, as a norm, belong to late stages of disease [45, 143].

Male Reproductive Organs

Secondary tumoral involvement of male genitalia is a very infrequent occurrence [7]. The *prostate* and the *seminal vesicles* are sometimes involved by lymphatic or venous spread from tumors of the pelvic district particularly, or the recto-sigmoid colon or the bladder [7, 146]. These lesions are generally voluminous, with an infiltrating margin, and without any specific structural feature [29, 146] (Fig. 84).

Metastatic invasion of the *penis* is relatively more frequent. In addition to the aforementioned primary tumors, prostate, renal cell, and bronchogenic carcinomas are also encountered [20, 147]. The pathway of diffusion is either through the lymphatic spread or retrogradely through the venous system, for malignancies originating in the urogenital and digestive tracts [7]. Hematogenous localizations are much rarer and secondary to distant malignanices [147]. Penile metastases predominantly originate in the cavernous bodies with a secondary, often asymmetric, priapism [147]. Invasion of the corpora spongiosa and urethra may also cause associated hematuria and dysuria [148]. Simultaneous cutaneous lesions in

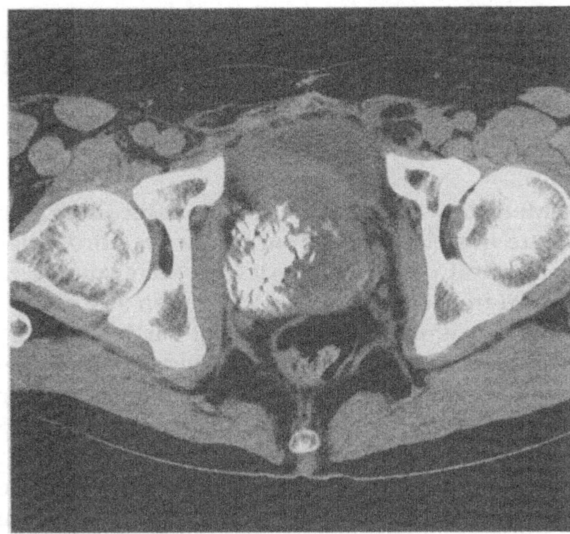

Fig. 84. Large secondary lesion of the prostate, with extensive calcifications, from *mucinous adenocarcinoma of the sigmoid colon*

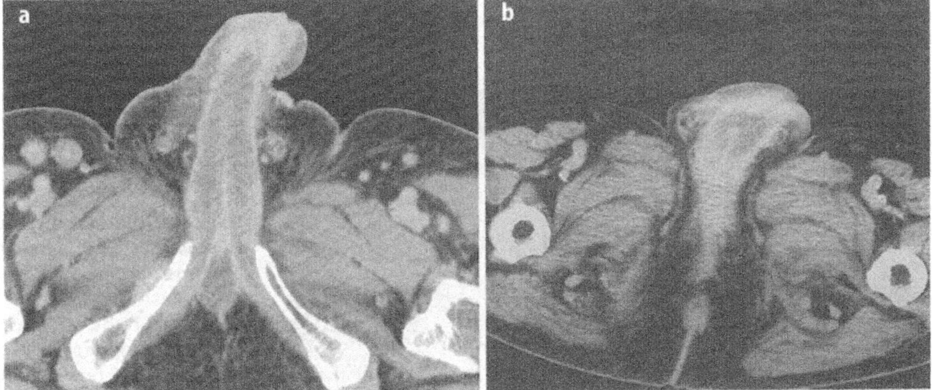

Fig. 85. a Penile metastasis from *sigmoid carcinoma*. The corpora cavernosa appear diffusely infiltrated by hypodense tissue. **b** Penile metastasis from *adenocarcinoma of the sigmoid colon*. Focal hypodense ill-defined lesion in a patient with La Peyronie's disease

the inguinal or pubic regions are frequently associated. The involved segment shows at CT diffuse or nodular hypodensity [29] (Fig. 85).

Metastatic involvement of the *testes* is also exceedingly rare, if we exclude leukemic and lymphomatous infiltrations. Testicular colonization is generally secondary to hematogenous diffusion from melanomas as well as prostate or bronchogenic carcinomas [20, 45]. These secondary tumors are multinodular and bilateral or demonstrate a diffuse infiltrative pattern of growth, and are often associated with hydrocele [149].

Similarly to what has been described in the vagina, retrograde venous diffusion is possible from those renal cell carcinomas causing neoplastic thrombosis of the left renal vein. In male patients colonization of the *epididymis* and *spermatic cord* occurs through the venous pampiniform plexus [1].

Soft Tissues

Metastatic localizations to soft tissues are an infrequent occurrence [20]. Both the striate muscles and the subcutaneous fibro-adipose tissue are relatively refractory to tumoral colonization, despite their volume preponderance in the body. Localization in these districts occurs often as a result of retrograde lymphatic diffusion from contiguous lesions [7, 29]. Particularly in the skeletal muscle, contractility, local pH variability, local lactic acid and other metabolite concentrations, local temperature, and increased intramuscular vascular pressure are all probably synergistic factors impeding neoplastic implantation [150, 151].

It is conceivable that *muscular metastases*, although infrequent, are underestimated in frequency since skeletal muscle is not routinely analyzed at autopsy. They are for the most secondary to melanomas, as well as colorectal, bronchogenic, mammary, and renal carcinomas [20]. The most frequently described locations include the diaphragm, iliopsoas, glutei, dorsal groups, and thoracic wall muscles [29, 150].

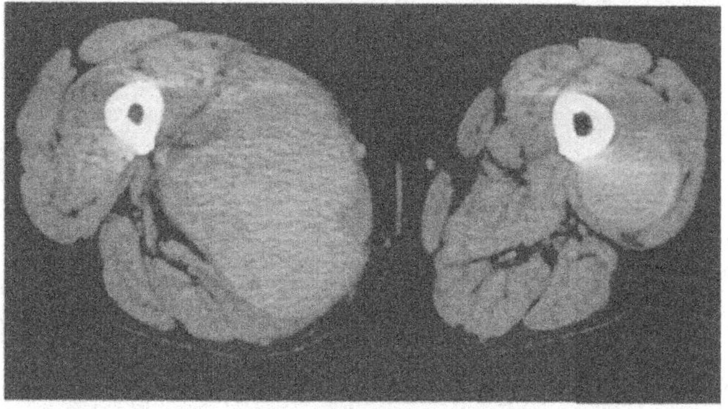

Fig. 86. Bilateral muscular metastases from a *mucoid adenocarcinoma of the lung.* Lesions in the vastus lateralis on the left and in the adductors group on the right, with heterogeneous density and contrast enhancement

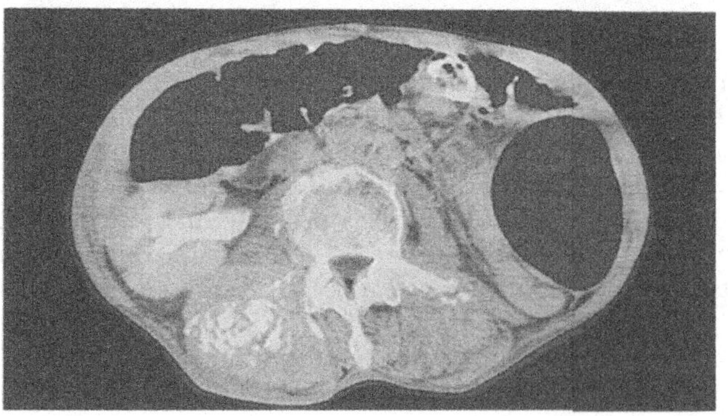

Fig. 87. Calcific involution of metastatic mass in the right paravertebral muscles from a *mucoid adenocarcinoma of the colon*

Computed tomography typically demonstrates an asymmetric enlargement of the muscular belly, associated with focal or diffuse hypodensity and occasional frank necrotic phenomena. These lesions are generally well delineated from the surrounding normal tissue only after intravenous administration of iodinated contrast [150]. Hypervascularity is a less frequent finding (Fig. 86). Calcific involution is also possible, especially in those lesions secondary to gastrointestinal mucinous malignancies (Fig. 87) [29]. The rare primary sarcomas are the main differential diagnostic entity at this level.

Subcutaneous lesions are, on the other hand, more frequently caused by hematogenous diffusion, although lymphatic spread may occur virtually anywhere [7, 152]. Again, melanomas, breast, lung, and renal cell carcinomas are the most frequent originating primary tumors (Figs. 88, 89) [20, 152].

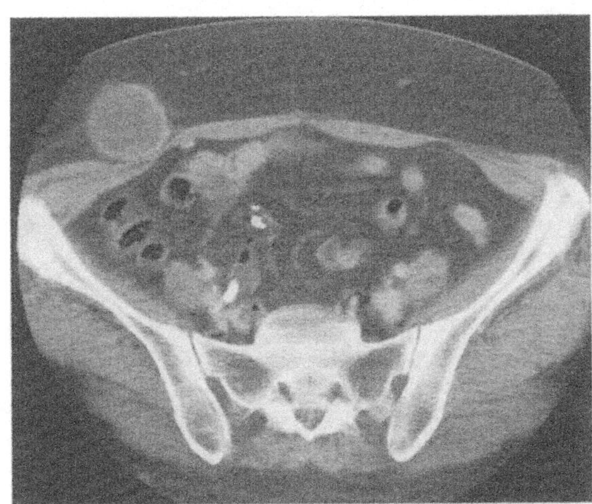

Fig. 88. Subcutaneous metastasis from *melanoma*

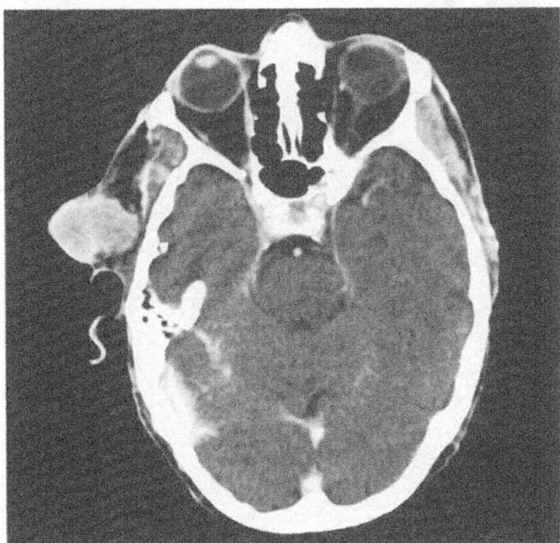

Fig. 89. Hypervascular subcutaneous metastasis from *melanoma*, located in the right pre-auricular and temporal region

The elevated contrast between the hypodense fatty subcutaneous tissue and the fluid or soft tissue density of the tumor makes these lesions very conspicuous [153], unless narrow fields of view are routinely employed, thus excluding large areas of subcutaneous tissue from visual examination. The differential diagnosis is versus sebaceous cysts, which, however, are generally more superficial and in close apposition to the cutaneous plane than the majority of metastases [152].

Bizarre Metastases

According to Wheelock and Frable [154], "bizarre" metastases are those located in dysplastic, malformed, or otherwise diseased organs, whether on a congenital or acquired basis (Figs. 85, 89–92). If most of the cases in this category represent little more than a curiosity, there are selected instances in which the preexistence of other pathologies may complicate or delay the correct diagnosis. For example, recent pathologic studies based on a dual series of Japanese and Italian patients affected by

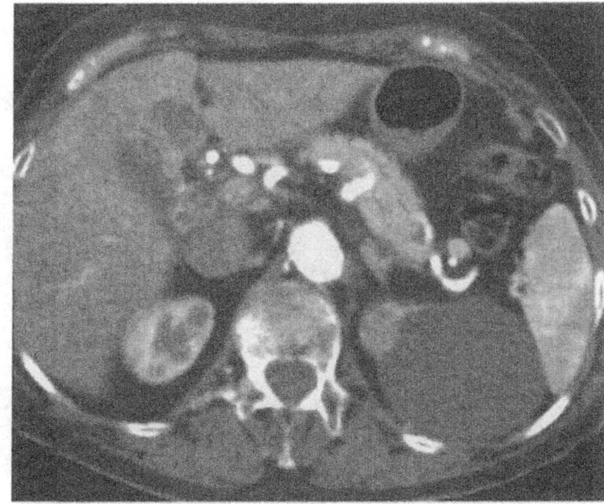

Fig. 90. Metastasis to the upper pole of the left kidney from a *small cell lung cancer.* There is an ipsilateral voluminous serous cyst

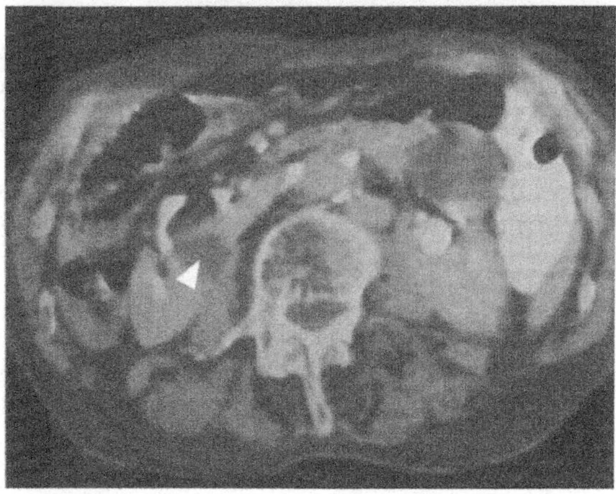

Fig. 91. Necrotic metastasis (*arrowhead*) from a *large-cell bronchogenic carcinoma* upon a horseshoe kidney, with a concurrent serous cyst on the left

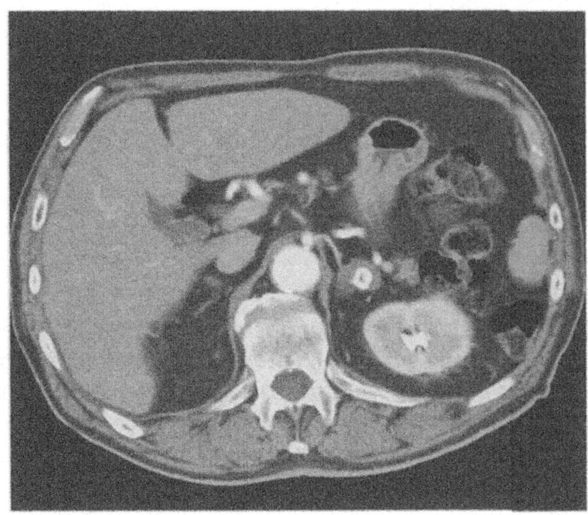

Fig. 92. Calcified metastasis from *mucoid adenocarcinoma of the colon*, upon a left adrenal adenoma

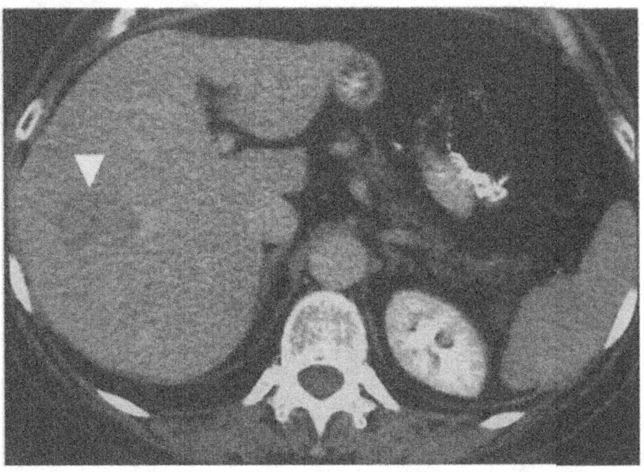

Fig. 93. Metastastic *colonic adenocarcinoma* (*arrowhead*) on a cirrhotic liver

hepatic cirrhosis [155] has documented metastatic lesions in approximately 15–20% of cases, several of which without knowledge of a preexisting malignancy (Fig. 93). Metastatic nature of focal lesions, detected at staging or follow-up of a neoplastic patient with concurrent hepatic cirrhosis, must always be considered, especially with concurrent suspicious lesions of other districts (gastrointestinal tract in the first place) and with suggestive biohumoral findings.

Differential Diagnosis Tables

The CT analysis of a lesion and correlation of its imaging findings with clinical history, physical findings and laboratory data are of paramount importance in a successful approach to the oncologic patient. With this in mind, we have attempted to create a series of tables which may offer a practical daily aid in the differential diagnosis of metastases. In each table any given lesion, its morphostructural features, and the possible synchronous metastases to other organs are all correlated to point toward a specific originating primary malignancy. This particular feature may be of help especially when the primary neoplasm is unknown or unsuspected.

Additionally, for each organ analyzed a few of the main imaging features of metastases have been correlated with their most frequent originating primaries. For reasons of space, only the organs' frequent site of metastatic diffusion is discussed. Additionally, analysis of unusual organs would be complicated by the extreme variability in appearance and by the multiplicity of tumors encountered.

Table 1a. Anatomic site of neoplastic colonization of liver

Morphology	Structure	Synchronous sites	Primary tumor
Macronodular	Pseudocystic, hypodense, ring enhancement, hypervascular	Nodes (para-aortic and mesenteric), peritoneum (ascites, carcinomatosis), ovary, adrenals, lung	Colon
Micronodular	Hypodense, ring enhancement, calcified	Nodes (celiac and gastrohepatic ligaments), peritoneum (ascites, carcinomatosis), ovary, lung (lymphangitic carcinomatosis)	Stomach
Micronodular	Hypodense, peripheral enhancement, pseudocystic	Lymph nodes (celiac, hepatic hilum, para-aortic), peritoneum (ascites, carcinomatosis), adrenals, lungs, pleura	Exocrine pancreas
Micronodular	Hypervascular, calcified	Nodes (celiac, hepatic hilum, para-aortic), peritoneum (ascites, carcinomatosis), adrenals, lungs, pleura	Endocrine pancreas
Macronodular	Hypodense, peripheral enhancement, pseudocystic	Lymph nodes (hila, mediastinum), bone, adrenals, pleura, cerebrum, kidney	Lung
Macronodular	Hypodense, peripheral enhancement, pseudocystic	Lymph nodes (celiac, hepatic hilum, para-aortic), peritoneum (ascites, carcinomatosis), lungs	Gallbladder
Micronodular	Hypervascular, sometimes hemorrhagic, calcified	Spleen, lung, intestine, brain	Melanoma

Table 1b. Structural characteristics of hepatic metastases

Calcified	Hypervascular – hemorrhagic	Cystic – pseudocystic
Mucinous carcinoma of gastrointestinal tract	Renal cell carcinoma	Ovarian carcinoma
Serous papillary or endometrioid ovarian carcinoma	Carcinoid	Colon carcinoma
Osteosarcoma	Colonic adenocarcinoma	Sarcoma
Chondrosarcoma	Breast Cancer	Breast Cancer
Endocrine pancreatic carcinoma	Melanoma	Pulmonary carcinoma
Melanoma	Endocrine pancreatic carcinoma	Pancreatic carcinoma
Mesothelioma	Sarcoma	Gallbladder carcinoma
Neuroblastoma	Leiomyosarcoma	
Medullary thyroid carcinoma	Pheochromocytoma	
Bronchogenic carcinoma		

Table 2a. Anatomic site of neoplastic colonization of lung

Morphology	Structure	Synchronous sites	Primary tumor
Micronodular, macronodular	Hemorrhagic	Bone, renal vein thrombosis, vena cava thrombosis, right atrium thrombosis, endobronchial, adrenal, brain	Renal cell carcinoma
Micronodular	Cavitary	Cervical nodes, pleural effusion	Head and neck cancer
Solitary macronodular	Pseudocystic, calcified	Liver, nodes (para-aortic, mesenteric)	Colon
Macronodular	Non-specific	Lymph nodes (retroperitoneal)	Testis
Micronodular	Non-specific	Lymph nodes (mediastinal), pleural effusion, bone, liver	Breast cancer
Micronodular	Calcified	Bone	Bone

Table 2b. Structural chracteristics of pulmonary metastases

Calcified	Cavitated
Osteosarcoma	Squamous cell carcinoma of head and neck
Chondrosarcoma	Squamous cell carcinoma of gastrointestinal tract
Mucinous papillary carcinoma of gastrointestinal tract	Sarcomas
Mucinous papillary ovarian carcinoma	
Medullary thyroid carcinoma	
Post-therapy evolution	

Table 2c. Morphologic characteristics of pulmonary metastases

Solitary nodule	Macronodular appearance	Lymphangitic diffusion	Miliary appearance
Colon carcinoma	Renal cell carcinoma	Lung carcinoma	Thyroid carcinoma
Melanoma	Wilms tumor	Breast carcinoma	Chorioncarcinoma
Sarcoma	Testicular carcinoma	Gastric carcinoma	Melanoma
	Osteosarcoma	Pancreatic carcinoma	Breast carcinoma
	Breast carcinoma	Colon carcinoma	Sarcoma
	Uterine carcinoma	Carcinoma of uterine cervix	Renal cell carcinoma
	Melanoma	Thyroid carcinoma	Gastric carcinoma
	Soft tissue sarcomas		

Table 3a. Anatomic site of neoplastic colonization

Morphology	Structure	Synchronous sites	Primary tumor
Nodular, supratentorial	Annular homogenous	Adrenal, bone, liver, lymph nodes (thoracic)	Lung
Nodular, infratentorial	Hemorrhagic	Bone, lung	Kidney
Nodular, supratentorial	Well-defined contours, ill-defined contours, hemorrhagic	Multiple viscera diffusely: lung, liver, bone, intestine, adrenal	Melanoma
Nodular, supratentorial, meningeal	Annular homogenous	Bone, liver, lung	Breast carcinoma

Table 3b. Structural characteristics of cerebral metastases

Calcified	Hemorrhagic	Cystic – pseudocystic
Mucinous carcinoma of gastrointestinal tract	Melanoma	Bronchogenic carcinoma
Serous papillary or endometrioid ovarian carcinoma	Renal cell carcinoma	Ovarian carcinoma
Osteosarcoma	Breast cancer	Colon carcinoma
Chondrosarcoma	Chorioncarcinoma	Breast cancer (after therapy)
Medullary thyroid carcinoma	Thyroid carcinoma	
Bronchogenic carcinoma		

Table 4a. Anatomic site of neoplastic colonization bone

Morphology	Structure	Synchronous sites	Primary tumor
Non-specific ■ Infrequent periosteal reaction ■ Rare soft tissue involvement *Most frequent locations* ■ Bony pelvis ■ Lumbar vertebrae ■ Proximal femoral epi- and metaphysis	Osteoblastic diffuse to focal	Pelvic lymph nodes	Prostate
Non-specific ■ Expansion of bone with frequent extension to soft tissues	Osteolytic	Lung, adrenal, liver, regional lymph nodes	Renal cell carcinoma
Non-Specific ■ Generally non-expansile *Most frequent location* ■ Spine and pelvis ■ Femurs	Osteolytic	Adrenal, brain, liver, mediastinal lymph nodes	Lung
Non-Specific ■ Frequent pathologic fractures ■ Frequent soft tissue involvement *Most frequent locations* ■ Bony pelvis ■ Vertebrae ■ Thoracic cage	Osteolytic Osteoblastic (rare)	Lung, pleura, mediastinal lymph nodes, liver	Breast
Non-specific ■ Frequent bony expansion *Ubiquitous involvement*	Osteolytic	Lung, regional lymph nodes	Thyroid

Table 4b. Structural characteristics of skeletal metastases

Osteoblastic	Osteolytic	Mixed
Prostate carcinoma	Pulmonary carcinoma	Breast cancer
Breast cancer	Breast cancer	Prostate carcinoma
Lymphoma	Renal cell carcinoma	Lymphoma
Carcinoid	Colonic adenocarcinoma	
Mucionous carcinoma of gastrointestinal tract	Thyroid carcinoma	
Pancreatic carcinoma	Bladder carcinoma	
Neuroblastoma	Colon carcinoma	
Medulloblastoma	Hepatocellular carcinoma Neuroblastoma Melanoma Ewing's sarcoma Osteosarcoma	

References

1. Morgan-Parkes JH (1995) Metastases: mechanisms, pathways, and cascades. Am J Roentgenol 164:1075–1082
2. MacDonald NJ, Steeg PA (1993) Molecular basis of tumor metastasis. Cancer Surv 16: 175–199
3. Nicholson GL (1993) Paracrine and autorcrine growth mechanisms in tumor metastasis to specific sites with particular emphasis on brain and lung metastases. Cancer Metastasis Rev 12:325–343
4. Liotta LA, Steeg PS, Stetler-Stevenson WG (1991) Cancer metastasis and angiogenesis: an imbalance of positive and negative regulation. Cell 64:327–336
5. Weiss L (1985) Metastastic patterns. In: Weiss L (ed) Principles of metastasis. Academic Press, London
6. Spremulli EN, Dexter DL (1983) Human tumor cell heterogeneity and metastasis. J Clin Oncol 8:496–509
7. Willis RA (ed) (1975) The spread of tumors in the human body. Butterworths, New York
8. Verschakelen JA, De Leyn P, Bogaert J, Baert AL (1996) Oncology imaging: nodal spread-intrathoracic nodes. Eur Radiol 6:251–261
9. Delorme S, van Kaick G [1996] Imaging of abdominal nodal spread in malignant disease. Eur Radiol 6:262–274
10. Park JM, Charnsagavej C, Yoshimitsu K et al. (1994) Pathways of nodal metastases from pelvic tumors: CT demonstration. Radiographics 1309–1321
11. Johkoh T, Ikezoe J, Tomiyama N et al. (1992) CT findings in lymphangitic carcinomatosis of the lung: correlation with histologic findings and pulmonary function tests. Am J Roentgenol 158:1217–1222
12. Herold CJ, Bankier AA, Fleischmann D (1996) Lung metastases. Eur Radiol 6:596–606
13. Spencer H (1977) Pathology of the lung (excluding tuberculosis). Pergamon Press, New York, pp 999–1010
14. Steiner H, Lammer J, Hackl A (1984) Lymphatic metastases to the esophagus. Gastrointest Radiol 9:1–4
15. Howell EJ, Lange EE de, Friedson HF Jr (1990) Linitis plastica of the colon: computed tomography findings. Gastrointest Radiol 15:69–71
16. Itoh T, Itoh H, Konishi J (1991) Lymphangitic liver metastasis: radiologic-pathologic correlations. J Comput Assist Tomogr 13:401–404
17. Wertheim I, Fleischacker D, McLahlin CM et al. (1994) Pseudemyxoma peritoneii: a review of 23 cases. Obstet Gynecol 84:17–21
18. Seshul MB, Coulam CM (1981) Pseudomyxoma peritonei: computed tomography and sonography. Am J Roentgenol 136:803–806
19. Caldemeyer KS, Mathews VP, Righi PD, Smith RR (1988) Imaging features and clinical significance of perineural spread or extension of head and neck tumors. Radiographics 18:97–100
20. Abrams HL, Spiro R, Goldstein N (1950) Metastases in carcinoma: analysis of 1000 autopsied cases. Cancer 3:74–85
21. Majoie CBLM, Hulsmans F-JH, Castelijns JA et al. (1993) Perineural tumor extension of facial malignant melanoma: CT and MRI. J Comput Assist Tomogr 17:973–975
22. Gaeta M, Volta S, Scribano E et al. (1996) Air-space pattern in lung metastasis from adenocarcinoma of the GI tract. J Comput Assist Tomogr 20:300–304

23. Ferrozzi F, Bova D, de Chiara F, Campodonico F, Bassi P (1995) CT of secondary neoplasms: unusual structural features. A pictorial essay. Clin Imaging 19:131–137
24. Wooten WB, Bernardino ME, Goldstein HM (1978) Computed tomography of necrotic hepatic metastases. Am J Roentgenol 131:839–842
25. O'Neill BP, Buckner JC, Coffey RJ et al. (1994) Brain metastatic lesions. Mayo Clin Proc 69:1062–1068
26. Ferrozzi F, Rossi A (1991) Aspect tomodensitométriques des metastases à forme calcifiante. J Radiol 72:305–312
27. van Zentan TEG, Golding RP, Taets van Amerongen AHM (1987) Osteosarcoma with calcific mediastinal lymphadenopathy. Pediatr Radiol 17:258–259
28. Maile CW, Rodan BA, Godwin JD et al. (1982) Calcification in pulmonary metastases. Br J Radiol 55:108–113
29. Ferrozzi F, Campani R, Garlaschi G (1997) La tomografica computerizzata nello studio delle metastasi: aspetti e sedi inusuali. Radiol Med 94:223–246
30. Ferenczy A, Talens M, Zoghby M, Hussain SS (1997) Ultrastructural studies on the morphogenesis of psammoma bodies in ovarian serous neoplasia. Cancer 39:2451–2459
31. Bernardino ME, Green B (1979) Ultrasonographic evaluation of chemotherapeutic response in hepatic metastases. Radiology 133:437–441
32. Chaudhuri MR (1970) Cavitary pulmonary metastases. Thorax 25:375–381
33. Zornoza J, Goldstein HM (1977) Cavitating metastases of the small intestine. Am J Roentgenol 129:613–615
34. Wright FW (1976) Spontaneous pneumothorax and pulmonary malignant disease: a syndrome sometimes associated with cavitating tumours. Clin Radiol 27:211–222
35. Dines DE, Cortese DA, Brennan MD (1973) Malignant pulmonary neoplasms predisposing to spontaneous pneumothorax. Mayo Clin Proc 48:541–544
36. Dodd GD, Boyle JJ (1961) Excavating pulmonary metastases. AM J Roentgenol 85:277–293
37. Husband JE (1996) Monitoring tumor response. Eur Radiol 6:775–785
38. Libshitz HI (1992) Metastases to the thorax. In: Greene B, Mum JR (eds) A categorical course in diagnostic radiology. Chest radiology. RSNA, Oak Brook, Illinois, pp 235–244
39. Peuchot M, Libshitz HI (1987) Pulmonary metastases disease: radiologic-surgical correlation. Radiology 164:719–722
40. Ptaszink R, McKenzie A, Hennesy O (1988) Cystic metastases from colon carcinoma. Australas Radiol 32:356–359
41. Shah HR, Love L, Williamson MR et al. (1989) Hemorrhagic adrenal metastases: CT findings. J Comput Assist Tomogr 13:77–81
42. Siskind BN, Malat J, Hammers L et al. (1987) CT features of hemorrhagic malignant liver tumors. J Comput Assist Tomogr 11:766–770
43. Swensen SJ, McLeod RA, Stephens DH (1984) CT of extracranial hemorrhage and hematomas. Am J Roentgenol 143:907–912
44. Salvolaine ER, Grecos GP, Howard J, White P (1985) Evolution of CT findings in hepatic hematoma. J Comput Assist Tomogr 9:1090–1096
45. Lee YN (1980) Malignant melanoma: pattern of metastases. Cancer 30:137–141
46. Lentini JF, Love MB, Ritchie WGM et al. (1986) Computed tomography in retroconversion of hepatic metastases from immature ovarian teratoma. J Comput Assist Tomogr 10:1060–1062
47. Palestro CJ, Vega A, Kim CK et al. (1990) Infected hepatic metastases. Role of In-111 leukocyte scintigraphy. Clin Nucl Med 15:434–437
48. Cascino TL (1993) Neurologic complications of systemic cancer. Med Clin North Am 77:265–278
49. De Clerck YA, Shimada H, Gonzales-Gomew I, Raffel C (1993) Tumoral invasion in the central nervous system. J Neurooncol 18:111–121
50. Hilal S, Chang C (1978) Specificity of computed tomography in the diagnosis of supratentorial neoplasms: consideration of metastasis and meningiomas. Neuroradiology 16:537–539
51. Jelinek J, Smirniotopoulos JG, Parisi JE, Kanzer M (1990) Lateral ventricular neoplasms of the brain: differential diagnosis based on clinical, CT and MR findings. Am J Roentgenol 11:567–574

52. Shiino A, Ito R, Nakasu S, Handa J (1998) Metastatic adenocarcinoma presenting as a homogeneously high-density mass on CT. J Comput Assist Tomogr 22:130–132
53. Chamberlain MC (1995) A review of leptomeningeal metastases in pediatrics. J Child Neurol 10:191–199
54. Coppage L, Shaw C, Curtis AM (1987) Metastatic disease to the chest in patients with extrathoracic malignancies. J Thorac Imaging 2:24–37
55. Hirakata K, Nakata H, Nagakawa T (1995) CT of polmonary metastases with pathologic correlation. Ultrasound CT and MRI 16:379–394
56. Crow J, Slavin G, Kreel (1981) Pulmonary metastases: a pathologic and radiologic study. Cancer 47:2595–2602
57. Davis SD (1991) CT evaluation for pulmonary metastases in patients with extrathoracic malignancies. Radiology 180:1–12
58. Gaeta M, Volta S, Stroscio S et al. (1992) CT "halo-sign" in pulmonary tuberculoma. J Comput Assist Tomogr 16:827–828
59. Hruban RH, Zerhouni EA, Wheeler PS et al. (1987) Radiologic-pathologic correlation of the CT halo-sign in invasive pulmonary aspergillosis. J Comput Assist Tomogr 11:534–536
60. Hirakata K, Nakata H, Haratake J (1993) Appearance of pulmonary metastases on high-resolution CT scans: comparison with histopathologic findings from autopsy specimens. Am J Roentgenol 161:37–43
61. Brown MJ, Miller RR, Muller NL (1994) Acute lung disease in the immunocompromised host: CT and pathologic examination findings. Radiology 190:247–254
62. Braman SS, Whitcomb ME (1975) Endobronchial metastasis. Arch Intern Med 135:543–547
63. Mahfouz AE, Hamm B, Mathieu D (1996) Imaging of metastases to the liver. Eur Radiol 6:607–614
64. Baker ME, Pelley R (1995) Hepatic metastases: basic principles and implications for radiologists. Radiology 197:329–337
65. Baron RL (1994) Understanding and optimizing use of contrast material for CT of the liver. Am J Roentgenol 163:323–331
66. Freney PC, Nghiem HV, Winter TC (1995) Helical CT during arterial portography: optimization of contrast enhancement and scanning parameters. Radiology 194:83–90
67. Rotondo A, Brunese L, Del Viscovo L (1996) Fegato e vie biliari. In: Pozzi-Mucelli R (ed) Trattato Italiano di Tomografia Computerizzata. Casa Editrice Idelson, Napoli, pp 917–971
68. Hughes JJ, Pollock WS, Schworn CP (1984) Branching pattern in CT of mucin-producing carcinoma of the liver. J Comput Assist Tomogr 8:553–555
69. Fishman EK, Kuhlman JE, Schuster LM et al. (1990) CT of malignant meloma of the chest, abdomen and musculo-skeletal system. Radiographics 10:603–620
70. Bernardino ME, Erwin BC, Steinberg HV et al. (1986) Delayed hepatic CT scanning: increased confidence and improved detection of hepatic metastases. Radiology 159:71–74
71. Bressler EL, Alpern MB, Glazer GM et al. (1987) Hypervascular hepatic metastases: CT evaluation. Radiology 162:49–51
72. Rossi A, Ferrozzi F, Rossi G (1990) La TC nello studio del surrene. Tipolitografia Benedettine, Parma
73. Greene KM, Brantly PM, Thompson WR (1985) Adenocarcinoma metastatic to the adrenal gland simulating myelolipoma: CT evaluation. J Comput Assist Tomogr 8:820–821
74. Cedermark BJ, Ohlsen H (1981) Computed tomography in the diagnosis of metastases to the adrenal gland. Surg Gynecol Obstet 152:13–16
75. Ferrozzi F, Campani R, Garlaschi G, Campodonico F (1997) Linfomi con localizzazione extranodale: aspetti con tomografia computerizzata e diagnostica differenziale. Radiol Med 94:429–441
76. Ha HK, Jung Ji, Lee MS et al. (1996) Differentiation of tuberculous peritonitis and peritoneal carcinomatosis. Am J Roentgenol 167:743–748
77. Ferrozzi F, Bova D, de Chiara F, Garlaschi G, Draghi F, Cocconi G, Bassi P (1998) Thin section CT follow-up of ovarian metastatic carcinoma: correlation with levels of CA-125 marker and clinical history. Clin Imaging 22:364–370
78. Rieux D, Laufenburger A, Soulier A et al. (1985) Aspect tomodensitométriques de la maladie gélatineuse du péritoine. A propos de 5 cas. J Radiol 66:297–302

79. Oliphant M, Berne AS, Meyers MA (1993) Spread of disease via the subperitoneal space: the small mesentery. Abdom Imaging 18:109–116
80. Oliphant M, Berne AS, Meyers MA (1993) Bidirectional spread of disease via the subperitoneal space: the lower abdomen and left pelvis. Abdom Imaging 18:117–125
81. Nywayama G (1998) Frequency and distribution of skeletal metastases. In: Resnick D, Nywayama G (eds) Diagnosis of bone and joint disorders. Saunders, Philadelphia
82. Soderlund V (1996) Radiological diagnosis of skeletal metastases. Eur Radiol 6:587
83. Jacobsson H, Goransson H (1991) Radiological detection of bone and bone marrow metastases. Med Oncol 8:253–261
84. Harrington KD (1993) Metastatic tumors of the spine: diagnosis and treatment. J Am Acad Orthop Surg 1:76–85
85. Coleman RE, Rubens RD (1987) The clinical course of bone metastases from breast cancer. Br J Cancer 55:61–66
86. Henriksson C, Haradsson G, Aldenborg F (1992) Skeletal metastases in 102 patients evaluated before surgery for renal cell carcinoma. Scand J Urol Nephrol 26:363–369
87. van den Brekel MW, Castelijns JA, Snow GB (1996) Imaging of cervical lmyphadenopathy. Neuroimaging Clin North Am 6:417–434
88. Ikezoe J, Kadowaki K, Morimoto S (1990) Mediastinal lymphnode metastases from non-small cell bronchogenic carcinoma: re-evaluation with CT. J Comput Assist Tomogr 14:340–344
89. Seely JM, Mayo IR, Miller RR, Muller NL (1993) T1 lung cancer: prevalence of mediastinal nodal metastases and diagnostic accuracy of CT. Radiology 186:129–132
90. Einstein DM, Singer AA, Chilcote WA, Desai RK (1991) Abdominal lymphadenopathy: spectrum of CT findings. Radiographics 11:457–472
91. Giron J, Chisin R, Paul JL et al. (1996) Multimodality imaging of cervical adenopathies. Eur J Radiol 21:159–166
92. Jager N, Weissbach L, Bussar-Maatz R (1994) Size and status of metastases after induction chemotherapy of germ-cell tumors. Indication for salvage operation. World J Urol 12:196–199
93. Ferrozzi F, Bova D, Campodonico F, Passari A, de Chiara F, Bassi P (1997) Pancreatic metastases: CT assessment. Eur Radiol 7:241–245
94. Max MB, Deck MDF, Rottemberg DA (1981) Pituitary metastasis: incidence in cancer patients and clinical differentiation from pituitary adenoma. Neurology 31:998–1002
95. Teears R, Silverman EM (1975) Clinicopathologic review of 88 cases of carcinoma metastatic to the pituitary gland. Cancer 36:216–220
96. Mukherji SK, Weeks SM, Castillo M, Yakaskas BC, Krishnan LA, Schiro S (1996) Squamous cell carcinomas that arise in the oral cavity and tongue base: Can CT help predict perineural or vascular invasion? Radiology 198:157–162
97. Arkas A, Bescos S, Raspall G et al. (1996) Perineural spread of epidermoid carcinoma in the infraorbital nerve: base report. J Oral Maxillofac Surg 54:520–522
98. Chong VFH, Fan YF, Khoo JBK (1996) Nasopharyngeal carcinoma with intracranial spread: CT and MR characteristics. J Comput Assist Tomogr 20:563–569
99. Ferry AP, Front RL (1974) Carcinoma metastatic to the eye and orbit: a clinicopathologic study of cases. Arch Ophthalmol 92:276–286
100. Green S, Som PM, Lavagnini PG (1995) Bilateral orbit metastases from prostate carcinoma: case presentation and CT findings. Am J Neuroradiol 16:417–419
101. Nakhjavani MK, Gharib H, Goellner JR, van Heerden JA (1997) Metastasis to the thyroid gland. A report of 43 cases. Cancer 79:574–578
102. Ferrozzi F, Campodonico F, de Chiara F et al. (1997) Metastasi tiroidee: aspetti con ecografia e tomografia computerizzata. Radiol Med 94:214–219
103. Shimaoka K, Sokal JE, Pickren J (1962) Metastatic neoplasms in the thyroid gland: pathological and clinical findings. Cancer 15:557–565
104. Som PM, Brandwein M (1996) Salivary glands. In: Som PM, Curtin HD (eds) Head and neck imaging, vol 2. Mosby, St. Louis, pp 1456–1459
105. Klatt EC, Heitz DR (1990) Cardiac metastases. Cancer 65:1456–1459
106. Tamura A, Matsubara O, Yoshimura N et al. (1992) Cardiac metastasis of lung cancer. A study of metastatic pathways and clinical manifestations. Cancer 70:437–442

107. McCrea ES, Jognson C, Haney PJ (1983) Metastases to the breast. Am J Roentgenol 141: 685–690
108. Vergier B, Trojani M, Mascarel I de (1991) Metastases to the breast: differential diagnosis from primary breast carcinoma. J Surg Oncol 48:112–116
109. Belton AL, Stull MA, Grant T, Shepard MH (1997) Mammographic and sonographic findings in metastatic transitional cell carcinoma of the breast. Am J Roentgenol 68:511–512
110. Iwaszkiewicz K (1995) Metastases to the breast: report of three cases. Eur Radiol 5:572–574
111. Soo MS, Williford ME, Elenberger CDE (1995) Medullary thyroid carcinoma metastatic to the breast: mammographic appearance. Am J Roentgenol 165:65–66
112. Ferrozzi F, Rossi A (1988) Gallbladder metastasis: CT appearance. Rays 13:23–25
113. Goldstein HM, Beydoun MT, Dodd GD (1977) Radiologic spectrum of melanoma metastatic to the gastrointestinal tract. Am J Roentgenol 129:605–612
114. Phillips G, Pochaczevsky R, Goodman J, Kumari S (1982) Ultrasound pattern of metastatic tumors in the gallbladder. J Clin Ultrasound 10:379–383
115. Charsangavej C, Whitley NO (1993) Metastases to the pancreas and peripancreatic lymph nodes from carcinoma of the right side of the colon: CT findings in 12 patients. Am J Roentgenol 160:49–52
116. Fugazzola C, Procacci C, Bergamo Andreis IA et al. (1990) Diagnostica per immagini delle metastasi pancreatiche. Radiol Med 80:559–675
117. Chowhan NM, Madajewicz S (1990) Management of metastases-induced acute pancreatitis in small cell carcinoma of the lung. Cancer 65:1445–1448
118. McLatchie GR, Imrie CW (1981) Acute pancreatitis associated with tumor metastasis in the pancreas. Digestion 21:13–17
119. Boudghene FP, Deslandes PM, LeBlanche AF, Bigot JM (1994) US and CT imaging features of intrapancreatic metastases. J Comput Assist Tomogr 18:905–910
120. Rumancik WM, Megibow AJ, Bosniak MA, Hilton S (1984) Metastatic disease to the pancreas: evaluation by computed tomography. J Comput Assist Tomogr 8:829–834
121. Berge T (1974) Splenic metastases. Frequencies and patterns. Acta Pathol Microbiol Scand 82:499–503
122. Marymont JH, Gross S (1963) Patterns of metastatic cancer in the spleen. Am J Clin Pathol 40:58–63
123. Rabushka LS, Kawashima A, Fishman EK (1994) Imaging of the spleen: CT with supplemental MR examination. Radiographics 14:307–315
124. Bruneton JN (1990) Metastases. In: Bruneton JN (ed) Imaging of gastrointestinal tract tumors. Springer, Berlin Heidelberg New York, pp 213–229
125. Caramella E, Bruneton JN, Roux P et al. (1983) Metatases of the digestive tract. Report of 77 cases and review of the literature. Eur J Radiol 3:331–338
126. Angelelli G, Macarini L, Fratello A (1987) Use of water as an oral contrast agent for CT study of the stomach. Am J Roentgenol 149:1084
127. Agha FP (1987) Secondary neoplasms of the oesophagus. Gastrointest Radiol 12:187–193
128. Anderson MF, Harell GS (1980) Secondary esophageal tumors. Am J Roentgenol 135:1243–1246
129. Green LK (1990) Hematogeneous metastases to the stomach. Cancer 65:1596–1600
130. Rodde A, Stines J, Regent D, Becker S, Conroy T, Weber B, Delgoffe C, Bour C (1987) Les pseudolinites gastrique d'origine mammaire. J Radiol 68:269–274
131. Ferrozzi F, Bova D, Garlaschi G (1994) Gastric metastases from retroperitoneal leiomyosarcoma: CT appearance. Abdom Imaging 19:298–300
132. Dick R, Pattison J (1972) Metastases to the stomach presenting as simple polyps. Br J Radiol 45:761–764
133. McNeill PM, Waginan LD, Neifeld JP (1987) Small bowel metastases from primary carcinoma of the lung. Cancer 59:1486–1491
134. Listrom MB, Davis M, Lowry S et al. (1988) Intussusception secondary to squamous carcinoma of the lung. Gastrointest Radiol 13:224–226
135. Kawashima A, Fishman EK, Kuhlamn JE, Schuchter LM (1991) CT of malignant melanoma: patterns of small bowel involvement. J Comput Assist Tomogr 15:570–574
136. Leidich RB, Rudolph LE (1991) Small bowel perforation secondary to metastatic lung carcinoma. Ann Surg 103:67–69

137. Antler A, Ough Y, Pitchumoni C, Davidian M, Thelmo W (1982) Gastrointestinal metastases from malignant tumors of the lung. Cancer 49:170–172

138. Krestin GP, Beyer D, Lorenz R (1985) Secondary involvement of the transverse colon by tumors of the pelvis: spread of malignancies along the greater omentum. Gastrointest Radiol 10:283–288

139. Ferrozzi F, Bova D, Campodonico F (1997) Metastatic disease of the kidney: CT findings. Sem US CT MRI 18:115–121

140. Ferrozzi F, Campodonico F, de Chiara F et al. (1993) Metastasi renali: aspetti TC e diagnostica differenziale. Eido Electa 4:161–167

141. Shirkhoda A (1986) Computed tomography of perirenal metastases. J Comput Assist Tomogr 10:435–438

142. Canozzi R, Benzi E, Santini D (1995) Metastasi ureterale da carcinoma mammario lobulare. Rara causa di urinoma. Radiol Med 90:158–160

143. Mazur MT, Hsueh S, Gersell DJ (1984) Metastases to the female genital tract. Analysis of 325 cases. Cancer 53:1978–1984

144. Mata JM, Inaraja L, Rams A et al. (1988) CT findings in metastatic ovarian tumors from gastrointestinal tract neoplasms (Krukenberg tumors). Gastrointest Radiol 13:242–246

145. Ferrozzi F, Castriota-Scanderbeg A, Piazza N, Bova D (1993) Calcified ovarian metastases from mucinous carcinoma of the colon. Clin Imaging 17:17–18

146. Berman JR, Nunnemann RG, Broshears JR, Berman IF (1993) Sigmoid colon metastatic to the prostate. Urology 41:150–152

147. Aubert J, Dore B, Grange P et al. (1988) Métastase pénienne d'un cancer prostatique. J Urol 94:475–477

148. Kelleher JP, Ashpole R, Pengelly AW (1989) Penile plaque: a presentation of metastatic renal carcinoma. Br J Urol 64:428

149. Pienkos EJ, Jablokow VR (1972) Secondary testicular tumors. Cancer 30:481–485

150. Schultz SR, Bree RL, Schwab RE, Raiss G (1986) CT detection of skeletal muscle metastases. J Comput Assist Tomogr 10:81–83

151. Seeley S (1980) Possible reasons for high resistance of muscle to cancer. Med Hypotheses 6:133–137

152. Patten RM, Shuman WP, Teefey S (1989) Subcutaneous metastases from malignant melanoma: prevalence and findings on CT. Am J Roentgenol 152:1009–1012

153. Dunnick NR, Schaner EG, Doppman JL (1978) Detection of subcutaneous metastases by computed tomography. J Comput Assist Tomogr 2:275–279

154. Wheelock MC, Frable WJ (1962) Bizarre metastases from malignant neoplasms. Am J Clin Pathol 37:475–490

155. Melato M, Laurino N, Mucli E (1989) Relationship between cirrhosis, liver cancer and hepatic metastases. An autopsy study. Cancer 64:455–459

Subject Index

Page numbers in *italics* refer to illustrations

Abscess 28,33
adenoid-cystic, carcinoma 10,32
adrenal glands 43
– adenoma with metastasis *82*
– hyperplasia 44
– metastases *13, 15, 24, 42, 44*
AIDS, related tumors 25
amylase 70
amylasemia 71
anaplasia, cellular 11
angiomyolipoma 72,73
angioneogenesis, tumoral 3
angiosarcomas 22,66
architecture, cytologic of metastases 11
aspergillosis 33
astrocytoma 28
azygos, hemiazygos venous system 8

Basal membrane 3
Batson's plexus 5,8
bizarre, metastases 81
bladder 74
– metastases *74*
– transitional cell carcinoma *49*
bone 48
– differential diagnosis 89
– lytic/blastic character 49
– structure of metastases 90
– metastases *13, 25, 30, 49, 50, 51*
brain 27
– differential diagnosis 98
– extraaxial 28
– intraaxial lesions 27
– metastases *13, 14, 16, 28, 29*
breast 62
– carcinoma, metastatic *13, 15, 30, 31, 36, 38,*
  42, 50, 56, 58, 59, 69
– metastases *62*
bronchioloalveolar carcinoma 10, 18
bronchogenic carcinoma 6, 21, 27, 35, 37, 43,
  57, 61, 64, 72, 75, 77

Calcification, in metastases
– dystrophic 17
– metaplastic 16, *17*

– mucoid 18, *18*
– orthoplastic 14
– psammomatous 18
carcinoid *42, 66*
cat scratch disease 53
cavitation, of metastases 20
cecum, see colon
cerebrospinal fluid 9
cerebrum, see brain
cholangiocarcinoma 41
chondrosarcoma 16, *17*
chorioncarcinoma 22, 68
cirrhosis 82
coccidioidomycosis 33
colon, rectum and sigmoid 71
– carcinoma *14, 21, 24, 41, 53, 64, 76*
– mucinous adenocarcinoma *19, 34, 78,*
  82
– leiomyosarcoma *55*
– metastases *71*
colonization, intravascular 3
corpora spongiosa 76

Diabetes insipidus, from pituitary metastases
  56
diencephalon 55
diffusion, of metastases 5
– extravascular 10
– hematogeneous 7
– lepidic 10
– lymphangitic 6
– lymphatic 5
– perineurial 9, 57
– seeding 6
– thrombotic 10
digestive tract, see gastrointestinal tract
Douglas, pouch of 9, 46
dystrophic, calcification 17

Embolization, neoplastic 35
enchondral ossification 16
endobronchial metastases 34, *35*
epididymis 78
esophagus 67
– metastases *68*

Ewing's sarcoma   58
extravascular diffusion   3
eye   59

Gallbladder   62
– mucoid adenocarcinoma   *22, 48*
– metastases   *63*
gastrointestinal tract   67
genital tract
– female   74
– male   76

Heart   60
– metastases   *61*
hepatocellular carcinoma   *50*
histiocytoma, malignant fibrous
    retroperitoneal   *32*
histology, of metastases   11
histoplasmosis   33
hydroureteronephrosis   74
hypervascularization of metastases   12
hypothalamus-pituitary   56

Implantation   3
infratentorial lesions   28
intravascular colonization   3
intussusception   70
invasion, local neoplastic   3

Kaposi's sarcoma   69
kidney   72
– metastases   *6, 17, 73, 74*
– renal cell carcinoma   *13, 16, 24, 35, 36,
    38, 64*

Lachrymal   59
larynx   60
leiomyosarcoma   *69, 74*
lepidic diffusion   10
leptomeningeal, carcinosis   28
linitis plastica, metastatic   7
liposarcoma
– mixoid, metastatic to the lung   *6, 34*
liver   39
– contrast medium administration
    and enhancement   39, 41
– differential diagnosis   84
– hepatocellular carcinoma   *50*
– metastases   *7, 14, 15, 19 – 25, 39 – 43*
– structure of metastases   85
lung   29
– bronchogenic carcinoma and other
    primaries   *12-16, 29, 39, 41, 44, 62,
    73, 78*
– consolidation   34
– differential diagnosis   86
– embolism, neoplastic   35

– growth rate   32
– hemorrhage   32
– metastases   *6, 11, 13, 16, 17, 21, 31 – 36*
– morphology   32, 87
– – adipose   33
– – calcification   33
– – cavitated   33
– – endobronchial   34
– – lymphangitic carcinomatosis   *37, 36*
– – sterile, after chemotherapy   37
– solitary nodule   32
– structure   87
lymphangitic carcinomatosis   *6, 14, 36, 37, 43,
    64, 65*
lymphnode   51
– calcification   54
– cystic transformation after chemotherapy
    54
– dimensions   52
– enhancement   52
– extracapsular diffusion   53
– false negative, false positive   52
– infiltration of neurovascular bundles   54
– structure   52
– metastases   *20, 52-55*

Meckel's cave   57
mediastinum
– carcinomatosis   *53*
medulloblastoma
melanoma, metastatic   *23, 31, 40, 60, 61,
    71, 79*
meningi, metastases   28
mesenteric metastases
    (mesocolon mesosigma)   *11*
miliary appearance   30
mouth
– epidermoid carcinoma   *54*
muscle   78
muscular metastases   *78*

Nasal cavity   *68*
nasal fossae   57
neuroblastoma   28

Omentum, see peritoneum
– omental cake   46, *47*
orbit   57
orbital metastases   *58*
osteoblasts   49
osteoclast   49
osteosarcoma, metastastic   *17, 74*
osteoslerotic, metastases   49
ovary   76
– metastases   *76*
– primary ovarian neoplasms   *7, 18, 19, 25,
    46 – 48, 66*

Pancreas   63
– metastases   *14, 64*
– primary neoplasms   *24, 36, 73*
pancreatitis, acute   64
paranasal sinuses   57
parathyroid carcinoma   *28*
parotid gland   60
pathogenesis of metastases   3
penis   76
– metastases   *76*
pericardium, neoplastic seeding   8
perirenal space   72, *73*
peritoneum   8, 45
– chemotherapy effects   46
– metastases   *18, 46, 47*
– pseudomyxoma peritonei   *9, 9*
– seeding   9
pharynx   59
pheochromocytoma   22
pituitary gland   56
– metastases   *62*
pleura   8, 37
– metastases   *38*
– seeding   8
proptosis   58
prostate   76
– metastases   *77*
prostatic carcinoma   49, *51*
psammoma bodies   18
pseudomyxoma peritonei   9
pulmonary arteries, neoplastic embolization   *35*

Rectum, see colon
retroconversion, after chemotherapy   24, *25*

Salivary glands   60
salpinges   9, 75
sarcoidosis   37
schwannoma   22
scirrous carcinoma of the breast   70
sebaceous cyst   79

sella turcica   56
seminal vesicles   76
sigmoid, see colon
soft tissues   78
small bowel   69
– carcinoid   *42, 66*
– metastases   70
spermatic cords   78
sphenoid   56
spleen   65
– metastases   *66*
steatonecrosis of the peritoneum   46
stomach   68
– carcinoma   *11, 36, 43, 53, 55, 63*
– leiomyosarcoma   *55*
– metastases   *69*
– mucoid adenocarcinoma   *40*
structure of metastasis   11–28, 90–102
subcutaneous tissues   79, *79*

Target appearance of metastases in small bowel   70
testes   77
– embrionary carcinoma   *20*
thrombosis, neoplastic   8
thyroid   59
– metastases   *57, 60*
– papillary carcinoma   *25*
tongue   60

Ureter   74
urinary tract   74
urothelial neoplasms   74
uterus   75
– sarcoma   *21, 33*
uvea   59

Vagina   75
vascularization of metastases   12
vulva   75

Wirsung's duct   65

Made in the USA
Monee, IL
07 July 2026